"The Church teaches that the phy[...] eminently personal. This book intro[...] [...]y of fascinating and diverse persons in the profession of medicine. Readers will experience their sense of vocation, their love for their patients, Christ and the Church, and their vision for medicine. This book is enlightening and inspiring."

— **John F. Brehany, Ph.D., S.T.L.,**
Executive Director and Ethicist,
Catholic Medical Association

"*Heart Sounds* tells the stories of twelve physicians' personal and professional lives. Their Catholic faith focuses their lives and relationships with patients. Prayer and engaging in conversations with patients regarding their faith beliefs are integral to their vocation as doctors. I enjoyed the book immensely and recommend *Heart Sounds* be read and reread by everyone engaged in health care. *Heart Sounds* should be on every health care professional's book shelf!"

— **Clement P. Cunningham M.D., K.S.G.**

"*Heart Sounds: 12 Catholic Doctors* is both inspiring and delightful to read. In the Christian tradition, Christ is sometimes referred to as the Divine Physician who has healed a spiritually sick and fallen humanity by his life, death and resurrection. The stories of the 12 Catholic physicians whom you will meet in this monograph will remind the reader that the healing mission of Christ and his Church continues in the world today through remarkable and deeply spiritual physicians such as these men and women. In our contemporary American culture, many Catholic professionals separate their Catholic faith with its moral and social implications from their professional concerns. These 12 Catholic doctors are sterling examples of dedicated disciples of Christ who are trying daily to fulfill the Lord's instruction to be 'the salt of the earth' and 'the light of the world.'"

— **Most Reverend Robert J. McManus, S.T.D.,**
Bishop of Worcester

"In these days of commercialization and impersonalized medicine, it is reassuring to read how twelve physicians joined their faith and their professional commitments. This is Christian evangelization in its best sense. I shall recommend this book to my medical students and residents who will find in it inspiration and encouragement."

— **Edmund D. Pellegrino, M.D., M.A.C.P.**,
Professor Emeritus of Medicine and Medical Ethics,
Georgetown University

"As a Catholic medical student ardently trying to live out my own call, *Heart Sounds* is a beautiful testament of hope, trust in God, and faith in the Church. Identifying with the passions, joys, and sufferings that each physician experiences provides a solidarity that is a most inspiring read."

— **Natalie Rodden**, 2nd year medical student,
President, Catholic Medical Student Association.

"*Heart Sounds* is truly an inspiration to me. It reaffirmed my commitment to continue to have my faith inspire my daily work as a Catholic physician and a teacher and educator of medical students in a secular medical school. We face many challenges on a daily basis and it is truly uplifting to know that we are not alone in asking for God's grace to live our vocation in treating our patients as we would treat Jesus Christ. I will strongly recommend this book to medical students, residents and colleagues to encourage them in their journey to live the unity of life in their daily work."

— **Leonard P. Rybak, M.D., Ph.D.**, President,
Catholic Medical Association, Professor of Surgery,
Division of Otolaryngology, Southern Illinois University
School of Medicine, Springfield, Illinois.

"*Heart Sounds* is a beautifully and inspiringly written account of twelve devoted Catholic doctors dedicated to living their faith within the context of the science and vocation of medicine. Each story summarizes, not the life of a living saint, but the life of a man or woman committed to medicine founded on and deeply informed by faith. I found the book inspiring and edifying. Thank you for this book, it is much needed in our discussion of the reason for the Catholic Church's involvement in healthcare. It is a book which helps us understand what it means for Catholics devoted to the faith to be involved in the art and science of medicine. *Heart Sounds* makes it clear that faith and science are not enemies but necessary friends. The beautiful faith manifested by the subjects in this book makes it clear why the Catholic Church takes its roles in healthcare so seriously. Healing involves much more than physical health."

> — **Most Reverend Robert F. Vasa**,
> Bishop of Baker, Oregon

"*Heart Sounds* is a powerful reminder that the Catholic physician's art is a vocation, not simply a career. As that vocation becomes ever more countercultural in the 21st century, witnesses like the twelve doctors who tell their stories here, and those who will be inspired by them, will be increasingly important in defending the culture of life from the encroachments of its adversaries."

> — **George Weigel**, Distinguished Senior Fellow,
> Ethics and Public Policy Center, Washington, D.C.

"The crisis in healthcare today is due in large part to a loss of our authentic identity as physicians and medicine as a vocation. Political proposals for reforming healthcare delivery risk undermining the very foundation of the medical profession, the doctor-patient relationship, because as G.K. Chesterton said, 'We don't know what we are doing, because we don't know what we are undoing.' In *Heart Sounds*, we see what is at risk of being undone in the extraordinary stories of the lives and practices of twelve physicians, each with a remarkable commitment to caring for the sick with competence and compassion. Their lives exemplify the identity of the true physician and will inspire all who read this book to work for the renewal of healthcare in America, preserving the principles and values these men and women have sacrificed their lives to uphold for the welfare of the sick, suffering and dying."

> — **R. Steven White, M.D.**, Past President, CMA and
> Chair, CMA Health Care Policy Committee

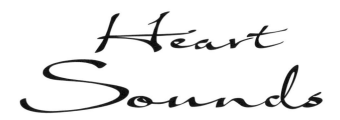

12 Catholic Doctors

Janice Steinhagen and John Howland, M.D.

St. Luke's Books
Southbridge, Massachusetts

First edition (2nd printing): 2010

ISBN 978-0-9845698-0-9

Available from:
Marian Helpers Center
Stockbridge, MA 01263

Orderline: 1-800-462-7426
Website: www.marian.org

The biblical quotations in this book, unless otherwise noted, are taken from the New American Bible, copyright 1986 by the United States Conference of Catholic Bishops.

To the memory of my father, Joseph Malego,
and to his patron, St. Joseph the Worker.

— J.M.S.

CONTENTS

ACKNOWLEDGEMENTS

Thanks to Fr. Kazimierz Chwalek of the Marians for getting us started. Bringing the project to fruition was the work of the Worcester Guild of the Catholic Medical Association. We thank the Guild's board of directors for their support. We would like to thank the executive director of the CMA, Dr. John Brehany, for his encouragement. Thanks to Fran Bourdon and the Marians for all the help with printing and promotion. Thanks also to Terese Karmel and Mary Gallagher for their painstaking editorial help, to Jennifer Kenning and Kathy Szpak for a beautiful design, and to our families for their patience. Finally, we would like to acknowledge and thank our Lord, Jesus Christ, to whom be all the praise and all the glory.

INTRODUCTION

Medical school is intense. One of the most striking and intense moments of my four years of medical school was in gross anatomy class. The professor reached into a jar of formaldehyde and handed me a human heart to examine. Located in the center of the chest, the heart is indeed a "vital organ." Yet the word heart connotes much more than the physical organ. We speak of the person with a "good heart" referring to their personality, their emotional nature, and their innermost inclinations. The "heart of the matter" is that which is central, the essence of something.

What is the sound of the heart? As the heart beats its valves open and close making sounds that can be heard with a stethoscope. Lub-dub, lub-dub, lub-dub, lub-dub. Each minute, 60-80 times, our hearts beat—lub-dub, lub-dub, 100,000 times a day. It's really quite an extraordinary fact to ponder. Even without a stethoscope, the heart sounds can be heard, but you must press your ear against the chest of another. It requires a degree of intimacy permitted to few. In 1816 it was René Laennec, a devout Catholic surgeon, living and working in the city of Nantes, who discovered that he could listen to the heart using a wooden tube, like an ear trumpet, a historical form of hearing aid.

This is a book about doctors, specifically about Catholic doctors. It is about what makes them tick, about their essence, their heart. Perhaps you, yourself, are a Catholic physician. You picked up this book, curious about some of your colleagues. Perhaps you are a nurse or other health care professional. Perhaps you are a college student thinking about a career in medicine or a medical student struggling with gross anatomy and wondering if you have made a big mistake. Perhaps you are thinking, "What is a Catholic physician?" Perhaps you are not Catholic, but just curious.

This is a book about 12 Catholic doctors, each with an interesting story to tell. These are real people telling the stories of their lives in their own words. The stories are about men and women, about family doctors and surgeons, about young doctors just starting their careers and those who are retired, looking back on their lifetimes. All told, these doctors have served the public for over 300 years. All of the doctors live and work within 50 miles of Worcester, Massachusetts but their stories take us all over the world, from Alaska to California, and from Korea to Ethiopia.

At the heart of each of these physicians are two things: a love for Jesus Christ and a love for the vocation of medicine. Medicine is or should be a calling, a vocation. The word "vocation" comes from the Latin word *vocare*, "to call." For some of us, faith and vocation are disconnected; there is little relation between what happens on Sunday morning at Mass and what happens Monday morning at work. Our society encourages this disconnect. These twelve physicians have each sought to integrate their Catholic faith and their vocation at the heart of their lives. This is a book about Catholic doctors, not doctors who happen to be Catholic. There is a difference.

We have chosen to focus on Catholic physicians but this is not to say that there aren't countless other physicians whom God has called to serve in the vocation of medicine. Most of the doctors in the book were born into the Church, but some were converts. All have come to see Christ as the center of their lives and are trying to live in the light of that reality. This is a book about the joy of a faithful life, but also about the challenges. Some of these physicians have received accolades for their actions; others have been maligned, even spat upon.

As many things do, this collection of stories started around a kitchen table. One evening several of us, physician members of the Worcester Guild of the Catholic Medical Association, were meeting at the home of Marie Romagnano, a nurse and founder of Healthcare Professionals for Divine Mercy. With us was Fr. Kaz Chwalek, a priest with the Marians of the Immaculate Conception. We were brainstorming, "How can we encourage Catholic physicians to integrate their faith and their vocation?" Inspired by the Holy Spirit, Fr. Kaz said simply, "Stories." The idea clicked and we were off and running.

In September of 2009 Janice Steinhagen, a talented writer, joined the project. A dozen Catholic physicians were chosen to be the subjects of the book. Between September and December Janice met with each physician, did an extensive interview, and drafted each chapter. The chapters were then edited and submitted to the physician for comment and approval. All patient names have been changed to protect confidentiality. Each chapter preserves the individual physician's voice, their manner of speaking, and their colloquial expressions. As a result the book is perhaps best heard rather than read and many no doubt will particularly enjoy the audio-version.

All of the doctors here are extraordinary but this is not a book about amazing or famous people. You are not likely to see them in the headlines or on television talk shows. These are unique, but not singular, individuals. Many communities have a Dr. Donovan or a Dr. Rollo. These are pretty ordinary people like you and like me. These are not perfect people, but men and women who struggle as we all do. Though ordinary and imperfect, each of these doctors is also remarkable. They are all remarkable for their compassion and dedication to the care of patients, something that is becoming less and less common in our era as medicine pursues an increasingly corporate and commercial agenda. Yet, as I'm sure each would freely admit, what's important about these stories is not what a few individuals have accomplished, but what God has chosen to do through them. Each would point to Jesus Christ as the substance and source of their accomplishments. Through faith, their lives have been transformed into something beautiful, something wonderful.

While most of the book is taken up with stories about medicine, we also are privileged to see how these men and women have lived their faith in their personal lives. We learn something of their lives of prayer and their relationships with God. We learn about their childhood and education, about their family lives, and about how they have personally dealt with illness and suffering. There's the psychiatrist who lovingly cared for her mother till God called her home at age 100 and the surgeon who along with his wife had three children and adopted seven more. There's the pediatrician who waited anxiously as his infant son underwent open-heart surgery and the internist who struggled to care for his patients while he himself struggled with prostate cancer. Through all this we begin to glimpse the essence of these unique individuals.

What does it mean to be a Catholic physician in our 21st century culture? Pope John Paul II described it as a culture of death with its embrace of abortion, utilitarian ethics, and euthanasia. Our culture is also dominated by a pervasive materialism and secularism. Our world does not accept the possibility of a transcendent God, of a spiritual reality, or of absolute truth. These are the stories of a few brave souls who have seen beyond the current fads to that deeper reality. These physicians have also recognized that they can't do it alone but must come together with other believers as part of the Church, the Body of Christ. And they have realized that they can't pursue their vocation in isolation from other Catholic physicians.

Many have found in the Catholic Medical Association an organization to call their own and to which they are called.

Most physicians are very private persons; we are trained to listen, not to speak. It is not a trivial matter to tell one's life story and bare one's heart, especially for a physician. We are deeply grateful to each of these twelve doctors who have so graciously agreed to be the subject of this collection of stories.

Finally, I think you will find much reason for hope in these pages—hope for the future. One of the "physicians" here is still a medical student, Rebecca Ackroyd, and one, Lori Warzecki, just finished her pediatric residency. Read their stories and you too will find reason for hope that God is raising up a new generation of Catholic doctors ready to serve Him in a profound new way.

May the sounds of these twelve hearts refresh and challenge your soul—as they have my own.

John Howland, M.D.
Southbridge, Massachusetts
Feast of St. Ignatius of Loyola
July 31, 2010

1

Dr. Lori Warzecki

THE GLORY GOES TO GOD

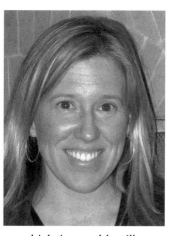

I love being a doctor. For me, it's the best profession in the world because it lets me be part of the healing that God does.

I grew up in Ludlow, Massachusetts, which is an old mill town. My dad is Polish and my mom is Portuguese and Irish. My parents and grandparents are very devout Catholics and very active in the Church. I went to public elementary school along with my identical twin sister, Lynn, and my younger sister, Lisa, but we attended CCD classes at church and almost all our extracurricular activities, like the Children of Mary, were church-related. My mom was one of the CCD teachers.

Lynn and I went to Cathedral High School in Springfield. Attending parochial school was an easy transition for me, since we had an active faith life at home. I loved Cathedral High, especially the daily Mass. I loved offering my day to God and asking Him to walk with me every day in class. Even when we had a day off from school, my mom and sister and I would go to Mass somewhere.

When we were teenagers, my parents signed us up as volunteer Candy Stripers at Ludlow Hospital. Every week we'd visit a couple of rooms at the hospital to feed the elderly patients. From an early age, Lynn knew that she wanted to be a nurse working in pediatric oncology. I also knew that I wanted to do something in health care but for a long time I wasn't sure what avenue to take, whether I wanted to be a pharmacist, a nurse, or a physician.

Lynn went right to nursing school. I spent four years taking community college courses part-time. I took one semester of nursing too, but found out that I cared more about what the doctor was doing than I did about giving the daily sponge baths. Nursing is important, but I could see that my own passion was trying to understand the patient's medical history and how the doctor's plan of treatment would help. So I dropped out of nursing. By that time, I was 23 years old. Since my age made me qualify as a non-traditional student, I was able to apply to a number of women's colleges that had scholarships for older students. But I was still uncertain what course my life was going to take.

One day I went to the Eucharistic adoration chapel in our parish church in Ludlow, Christ the King, and prayed, "Lord, I give it to You. My sister's a nurse, and we're twins, but I feel that's not what you're calling me to do. If I get accepted into one of these colleges, just make it clear to me that that's the route I'm supposed to go. It's not about what I want, but what You want."

God did make it clear and I was accepted at Wellesley College where I majored in biochemistry/pre-med. I also started going on medical mission trips. The first trip took place during winter break of my freshman year, when I went to Panama with the group Christian Medical Missions International. It was my first time out of the country. I was given a list of precautions: Put the insect repellent permethrin on all your clothes, get a mosquito net to sleep under, don't bring any closed-toe shoes because there are lots of scorpions that hide in them, and be sure to shake out your sandals before you put them on.

When I told my parents these things, my dad said, "We need to go to the Army-Navy store." So we went shopping, and we bought all the things I "needed." When I look back on it now, I think, "Oh my gosh, how ridiculous!" I had two suitcases filled with stuff for my two weeks in the jungle. Now I go on trips with just a backpack and I'm fine.

My itinerary was to fly from Boston to Houston, where I was to meet the rest of the mission team, and then we were to fly to Panama. But I had used a travel agent who wasn't well versed in English and didn't know the airports in the United States. She flew me to Houston's Hobby Airport (the domestic airport) and then I was to fly from Houston Intercontinental to Panama. But the agent didn't know that they were two different airports and since I had never traveled away from the East Coast, neither did I.

After I arrived at Hobby Airport, I looked all over for the international flights, but I didn't see anything. When I inquired, I was told that Intercontinental Airport was about 45 minutes away. So I hopped into a taxi. When we pulled up at the terminal and I asked the driver how much the fare was, he asked me "How much do you have?" I was kind of naïve, so I told him I had $45—and of course he said, "That's exactly what it'll be!" So he took all my money but I didn't care; I just wanted to get to Panama.

Going through security, my belt buckle set off the metal detector and I had to go back through a second time. Then somebody stole my Wellesley sweatshirt off of the conveyor belt, the sweatshirt that I had so proudly worn (maybe too proudly) because I'd gotten a scholarship. After finally clearing security, I ran and reached my gate just as the door was closing. I frantically spoke to the agent who said, "Oh, your party left a letter for you." The letter read, "Sorry we missed you, maybe you can join us on our next trip." I begged the agent to let me board the plane—it hadn't yet left the gate—and she let me on. This was before the tightened security at airports. I'm sure I would never be allowed to do it now.

I was out of breath, but I made it! As the plane took off and headed south, I sat there, panting. After I had finally relaxed, I realized, "My luggage...!"

So in spite of all the planning and trips to the Army-Navy store, I arrived in Panama without any of the things "necessary" for a medical mission in the jungle. But it was an opportunity for God to show me that all I really needed was within. In creating me, He had already equipped me for this job.

Once we had arrived in Panama, the other volunteers told me, "This is an opportunity for us to share with you, to help a sister and a colleague." So they opened up a pack of WalMart underwear and gave me a couple of pairs and cut one of their own mosquito nets in half. My luggage didn't arrive until we were about to leave for home but by then I had learned to trust in God, not in the permethrin-sprayed mosquito net from the Army-Navy store.

On that first mission trip, I held flashlights for dentists and worked in the pharmacy, and I loved it. I thought, "This is really cool. I definitely want to be a doctor and come back as a medical missionary." I really felt that the Lord was leading me. He had brought me to the mission field and said, "These are the plans I have for you." Even so, I kept praying for the Lord's help and guidance. I was still an undergrad and I wasn't sure I could get into medical school.

That summer following my trip to Panama, I went to Guatemala with Habitat for Humanity to build houses for the Mayans. Later, I went with CMMI to Nicaragua. From then on, for most of my breaks from college, I'd come home and see my parents briefly, then fly out of Boston or Hartford to a medical mission. In the years since that first trip to Panama I have been on over 30 mission trips to countries all over the world. My travels have taken me to all the countries of Central America and to Peru, Ecuador, Venezuela, Columbia, and Brazil in South America. I have done mission work in Israel, Palestine (Gaza), Jordan, and Egypt. I was in Pakistan after the earthquake in 2005 and in Haiti following the terrible earthquake this year. I have worked in China, India, and Indonesia and served in a number of countries in Africa, including Ghana, Liberia, Ethiopia, Kenya, Sudan, and Zambia. Many of my early trips were with Medical Ministry International. My recent work has been with World Medical Mission (Samaritan's Purse), Hands of Mercy, and E3 Partners.

During my second year at Wellesley, I decided to change my major to Spanish. My advisor said, "You're crazy! You should stay in science. What if you don't get into med school?" But when I was in Panama, I couldn't really talk with any of the people. I saw missionaries fluent in Spanish who could take patient histories and, just as importantly, cry with their patients because they understood them. With a translator, things are lost. I left the advisor's office that day feeling that God was telling me I needed to be fluent in Spanish. So, instead of listening to my advisor, I changed my major and went to Spain to study abroad. There I discovered it's one thing to learn conversational Spanish, but medical Spanish is a whole different thing. From the library I took out books on medical Spanish and studied all the specialized vocabulary. Eventually when I went on mission trips, instead of just holding flashlights, I was able to translate for the doctors. My first translating mission was with Medical Ministry International in Ecuador. After that, on my college breaks, I went to a number of Spanish-speaking countries.

After a big hurricane in El Salvador in 1998, a Protestant missionary organization emailed me that they needed a Spanish translator, so I went to help them. That mission challenged me because the team was very, *very* Protestant. On Ash Wednesday, when I was asking about where I could receive ashes, they said, "You're a *Catholic*? When are you going to come to know Jesus?" I said, "But I do know him!" In a way, they seemed so much more Christian than I, because they could quote Scripture so freely. I think they wanted me to go up at altar call and convert from Catholicism to their brand of Christianity. But I didn't see it as about that. I don't put God or Christianity into a box like that. All the different denominations are man-made; I don't see denominations in the Bible.

Even so, I grew in that situation because seeing them as "more Christian" helped make me stronger. It made me question my own faith and ask important questions such as: were they "more Christian" because of some aspect of their living and their interactions with each other? They helped me to see that I wasn't serving others with my whole heart. The whole experience really made me examine where I was in my walk with Christ, how much I depended on Him, and how much I saw Him as my Savior.

After I finished Wellesley, I had some interviews, but I didn't get into medical school right away. I thought maybe my advisor was right, that I should have stayed a science major. So I applied for a research position in a lab at the University of Massachusetts Medical School. I worked there for more than two years while I prepared for the Medical College Admission Test. We were doing research on Huntington's disease, a hereditary and fatal neurologic disorder. But at the same time, I was also volunteering at St. Anne's Free Medical Clinic, which served many Hispanic immigrants, making my knowledge of Spanish helpful. Volunteer work there really encouraged me to pursue med school and clinical medicine. The doctor in charge of the Clinic, Dr. Clermont, really encouraged my interest in medical missions.[1]

A number of the other docs at St. Anne's were from the University of New England, an osteopathic school. Osteopathy is very holistic. In addition to the standard medical history, they took spiritual histories and they really seemed to know what was going on at multiple levels with their patients. I also learned that UNE had a good Catholic community and a chapter of the Christian Medical and Dental Association (CMDA) on campus. So it was pretty natural that I would apply there. Thankfully, I was accepted.

I spent four years at the University of New England Medical School, which is in Maine. I was active with CMDA there, and through it I heard about a program called In His Image (IHI), a Christian family practice residency in Tulsa, Oklahoma. The program trains doctors to really recognize the gifts God has given them and to apply their knowledge and abilities to glorify Him. They see medicine, whether at home or in the mission field, as a calling, not just a job.

I contacted IHI and kept in touch all through med school, although I actually struggled with the idea of going there for my

---

1. Dr. Harvey Clermont is the subject of Chapter 7 of this book.

residency. I was drawn to them because of all the medical mission work they do. But they are a family practice residency and I didn't feel drawn to the geriatric part of family practice. I prayed, "God, I know You're calling me to do medical mission work. What better place to train than a place where physicians actively do that as part of the curriculum?" Finally, after much prayer, I decided to list them as my first choice. On Match Day I was given a position at In His Image.[2]

The next year was wonderful and challenging. Growing up Catholic, I wasn't used to praying out loud. I'd say to friends, "I'll pray for you," and most of the time I did. But in medical school, when I was wearing a white coat, I was afraid the hospital would kick me out if I asked a patient, "Can I pray with you?" However, at In His Image, the physicians, most of whom were Protestant, were comfortable with praying out loud. They had a long-standing good relationship with the hospital where they trained. People knew they were Christian physicians, offering something different to patients, and they respected that.

I've always considered myself to be a devout Catholic, but I'm a Christian too. When I was at IHI in Tulsa, my faith was tested—not in a bad way, but as if to tell me, "Lori, stand up for what you believe. It's not so different from what they believe. You're all Christians." That experience helped me really embrace my faith and be outspoken in expressing it. I prayed, "Okay, God, I will speak up for you. I won't be intimidated."

One of my patients was a young man named Antonio who had leukemia.[3] He had come illegally from Mexico to work in the United States and was sending money back home to his family. He was partying one night and passed out. He thought it was from drinking, but after he passed out several more times, he finally came to the hospital.

When we realized Antonio had leukemia, I thought, "Do I tell him this news? What do I do? It's so sad that his parents aren't here. He's not going to have anyone with him when he gets the news that he has cancer and the treatment will be very difficult

2. The Match is a competitive process for placing students in residency training programs after medical school. Students from around the country submit a list of their choices and the residency programs also submit a list of preferred applicants in rank order. Using a computer algorithm the two lists are matched. On Match Day, the third Thursday of March each year, the results are announced in ceremonies at medical schools across the country.
3. Here and throughout the book, names of patients have been changed to protect confidentiality.

with an uncertain prognosis." Through my worries, God really spoke to me, "He is *not* alone, Lori! I am with him. If you say you're a Christian, and you say I am with you, like you always tell Me when you pray, how can you sit in front of a patient and think God is not with him?"

"All right, God," I said. "You *are* with him. I just have to help him realize this."

So I asked Antonio in Spanish, "Do you have any particular faith?" He told me he was raised a Catholic, but since he had left Mexico, he hadn't done anything with his faith. "God probably exists," he said, "but I just want to get better so I can make money to send back to my family, because they're poor."

I told him, "Well, it's going to be a bit of a rough road ahead. But God loves you. He is with you. He doesn't care that you haven't prayed in months, He just wants you to start seeking Him now."

Antonio broke down in tears. "So often, I wanted to go back to praying to God," he said. "But I've just been too bad since I left my family. I hang out with my new friends, we drink all the time, and we're with girls. I know what the Catholic faith taught me back in Mexico and what my mom and dad would say. Sometimes in my struggles here in America, I have thought about God, but I thought, 'I can't go back to praying. God's not going to listen to *my* prayers.'"

In his hospital bed that day, Antonio wanted to pray out loud. I thought, "Thank God someone wants to do that!" So he prayed in Spanish, asking God to be with him. He prayed, "I know I'm sick. I want to be well. I want you to forgive me for what I've done." Every day after that, part of my rounds with him included praying together.

During my time at In His Image, I grew in my faith and got comfortable talking about it. Every day in the hospital, the patients saw lots of staff members—respiratory therapists, people who drew blood, nurses—and the patients knew something was different when these people prayed for them. People of faith, especially, appreciated that. Prayer opens the door for people to realize that God is with them in their happy times in life, as well as in sickness and sad times. Sometimes, we as physicians can be at a place in people's lives where other people can never go. At IHI we were trained to take a spiritual history with each patient. Patients would often talk about where they were in their faith, about their struggles. They'd want to pray. I was surprised how often patients wanted that.

I still keep in touch with the doctors in Tulsa who trained me. They were mentors who cared so much about where patients and their families were spiritually. I would be busy rounding on a patient and mention that someone was a DNR,[4] and my attending would ask, "Where is that person in their faith, knowing they might not make it through the night? How is the family dealing with knowing they're going to lose a family member?"

The doctors at IHI trained me to be a Christian physician, not a physician who is a Christian. It's not "I'm wearing a white coat so the glory goes to me." The glory goes to God. If you say to a patient, "Well, the odds aren't good, but I'll pray for you," then when God does heal them, they remember: God answered those prayers. For some it's just exactly what they need; it plants a seed of faith in their heart. Patients would ask me, "Well, Doc, I got better! What made you pray for me that day?" I tell them, "It was God."

I try to remember that every patient I treat is divinely appointed by God for me to see. So I'm going to care for them as Christ would care for them. With every patient I always pray that Christ might be reflected through me. A mother once asked me, "Why do you take such an interest in my child, who has cerebral palsy and can't even talk back to you? People just see her as a nuisance with all her difficulties." I answered, "She's a special child of God. Yes, she has her challenges, but she means so much to God. He has a special plan for her life." I can really see that, so I tell patients that I'm a Christian physician, that I'm praying for them, and that prayer is just as important as writing a prescription for an antibiotic. Christ is the Great Physician. We're just His hands and feet.

In 2005, I traveled with IHI to Pakistan after an earthquake to work in a refugee camp. I had a limited visa, which only allowed me to do disaster relief in a restricted zone. Pakistan is a Muslim country and the authorities wanted to make sure we were not traveling around preaching the Gospel. Muslim Sharia law strictly prohibits Christians from sharing their faith. In the refugee camp the women didn't want to be seen by male physicians. I saw a woman who was pregnant and bleeding who had walked for days to get to the camp. This was a problem she would never tell a male doctor. I went up and down the rows of tents, tending to the women and also to their

---

4. A "Do Not Resuscitate" or DNR order states that cardio-pulmonary resuscitation (CPR) should not be attempted if a person suffers cardiac or respiratory arrest.

children. I really loved being with the children, many of whom had broken bones and other injuries because building materials or rocks had fallen on them in the quake.

After I returned from Pakistan, I grew more and more uneasy about continuing in family practice. I did a pediatric rotation and loved it. Throughout that rotation I prayed, "God, do you really want me to change to pediatrics?" I felt the answer was yes, so I told my residency directors at IHI that I felt called to leave their three-year program after just one year. They were wonderful about it; they had someone else who wanted to enter the program, so it worked out perfectly for both of us.

I transferred to the pediatric residency at Loma Linda Children's Hospital in California. It is a very busy children's hospital run by the Seventh-Day Adventists, with a high focus on missions. I didn't have any reservations; I knew God was calling me there. But I did wonder, "God, what is a Seventh-Day Adventist? Will they be okay with me being Catholic?" I remembered that In His Image had been evangelical Christian, and I had loved those doctors and learned so much from them. It turned out that Loma Linda was much the same. The staff included Seventh-Day Adventists as well as other Christians and there were always opportunities to pray with patients.

The pediatric residency was challenging. I had an 80-hour workweek, but I don't think it was ever just 80 hours. One of my patients, Lisa, was a teenager who had been thrown from a car in a motor vehicle accident, resulting in a severe brain injury. Her parents were still mourning the recent loss of their son, who had been the innocent victim of a gang shooting, and now their daughter was in a vegetative state.

Every day I'd go in to see Lisa, but her condition never improved. She had already been in the hospital a couple of months when I first saw her; other residents who had taken care of her had come and gone, and from their two-month-old notes I saw that she really wasn't making any progress. The neurosurgeon had told her parents that this was how Lisa was going to be. He told them they could choose to take her off the ventilator, but then she wouldn't breathe on her own and would die. Or they could choose to withdraw her feeding tube, and she would die of starvation and dehydration.

But Lisa's mom, who was Catholic, said she couldn't do either. "Lisa will live until God calls her home," she said.

Lisa's care was very complicated and it took me almost an hour every day. I didn't take the time to see where her mom was spiritually, as I would have at IHI. One day on rounds, I saw Lisa's mom in tears. "There's no change," she said. "She's my daughter. I have her cell phone and I look at the 400 texts she sent me that last month before the accident, and I think, this was my daughter. And now," she said, gesturing to the bed, "*this* is my daughter."

I broke down in tears too. This was so hard for her. I should have asked her about all this two weeks earlier, instead of now, when I saw her crying. We talked about faith. "These doctors want me to just give up on Lisa," she said, "but I know God hasn't given up on her, because I'm Catholic. This is what I believe, and what Lisa believes."

I asked her if we could pray together, and we prayed for Lisa. From then on, praying with her was the most important thing I had to do. I didn't care if that meant I had to get up early. For months we had been like robots going in and out of Lisa's room: Check the ventilator, it's leaking, we change this button. That's all. But it wasn't checking the ventilator that this mom needed; she needed love and prayer to assure her that someone cared about her daughter and that Lisa was really in God's hands.

When my rotation was finished, Lisa's mom didn't want me to go. Through her tears, she told me that I had been a blessing for her and that she could now give this situation to God in a way she hadn't been able to before. She thanked me for praying with her every day. "Every day, Dr. Lori, you would listen to Lisa. You put the stethoscope on her chest and you would rub her hair and say, 'Hi, Lisa. Hi, Lisa.' Most people were just in and out, doing this, this, and this." I attributed her gratitude to God in me, recognizing what she needed. I think that's something we can and should do as Catholic physicians and as Christians.

She gave me a CD of Lisa's favorite songs, which made me cry when I listened to it. Lisa was eventually transferred to a nursing home facility. I still keep in touch with the family and go to see Lisa there.

Then there was seven-year-old Robby, who was diagnosed with cancer when he was five or six and now, two years later, was in remission. He had even been featured in the Make-a-Wish Foundation's calendar. But he kept feeling that something was going to happen to him. We thought it might be a post-traumatic stress reaction since he was still going into the office for check-ups, and seeing all the bald kids with portacaths. Perhaps he thought he was still sick. He was actually referred to a psychologist because he kept saying he was going to die, even though he was in remission and doing fine.

One night at home, Robby asked his mom if he could sleep with her. When he'd lain down beside her, he asked, "Mommy, does Jesus look like He does in the pictures? When I go to heaven, how will Jesus know what I look like? How will He find me? Do I have to go look for Him or will He be there waiting for me?"

His mom said, "Oh, Robby, let's not talk about this. Jesus knows exactly what you look like. He even knows how many hairs you have on your head." She thought Robby was thinking he still had cancer. He asked her to put her hand over his heart, and they fell asleep like that.

A few weeks later, Robby's dad was at home with him when he heard a loud thump coming from upstairs. He ran up and found Robby unconscious on the floor. He initiated CPR and called 911. The ambulance brought Robby to the closest hospital, where I happened to be on call. We did CPR on him for hours, with plans to transfer him to Loma Linda if we could stabilize his heart rate.

I put in a central line and he was doing okay, but all of a sudden there was an irregular rhythm on the monitor. He went into cardiac arrest again, and we ended up doing CPR for another couple of hours. Through all that time, Robby's mom and dad were praying out loud. I noted that on his chart, and as I was doing the CPR I prayed too: "Please God, they're calling out to You. If it's Your will, let Robby live."

Robby did live. We stabilized his heart rhythm, put him on a ventilator, and transferred him to Loma Linda. For a whole month he lived on a respirator in the ICU, but he never even opened his eyes. I told his parents, "I heard you praying that night when Robby came in. I was praying for him too. Any time you want to pray together, I'd love to do that with you." So we did. I cared for Robby through the whole month.

In that time, his mom really opened up to me about what a struggle it was to see her son this way. "We'd gone through that whole cancer scare, not knowing if he would die, and we'd gotten over that," she said. "Robby was even on the Make-a-Wish calendar, as a kid who was going to make it. At least he could talk then—he was still Robby. Now he's hooked up to a ventilator, he's not even responding when you grab his hand. His baby sister at home is asking, 'Where's Robby?'"

The physicians at Loma Linda were great, but some of them had suggested to Robby's mom and dad that they should remove him from the breathing machine. The parents prayed about that a lot, and felt that God was telling them, "Trust Me. Take him off the machine, and if I want him to continue breathing, he will." When they finally removed him from the machine, nobody expected Robby to take a single breath. But he did. He continued to breathe, and his parents took him home. He's still living today and although he is neurologically devastated, there are some neuronal pathways reconnecting. They're doing hyperbaric therapies and other modalities for him. He now smiles when he hears his parents' voices.

I still keep in touch with Robby's mom and dad. When they found out I was doing a mission trip to Sudan, they brought me a box full of his toy cars from when he was little. They told me, "He may never play with these again if he stays in the state he's in. But even if he does wake up and realize all the toy cars he loved are gone, he'd be so happy that the kids in Sudan are playing with them, because that was Robby."

Oh my gosh, it felt like I was holding Robby in a box. Even though I was just a resident taking care of Robby, his parents had seen how much I cared about him. They told me, "We want to extend the care you gave him to the kids you're going to care for in Sudan." So I took Robby's toy cars to Sudan. The children didn't even know how to use toy cars; I had to show them.

I hope Robby's parents saw Christ in me. I really see my interactions with patients as a prayer: "God, I want them to see You through me." I don't mean to suggest in any way that I'm superior to anyone else. I am so not perfect! I'm just saying that I want to be used by God so people can see Him, so He can help these families. The more we love God, the more we allow ourselves to be used by God.

So many times in suffering, it's hard to see where God is. Moms will say that all the time: "How could God do this to my child?" And I say to them, "God's not punishing your child. Suffering is a part of all of our lives. We all have different crosses, different ways we suffer."

I was in medical school when I first went to Ghana with CMMI, as a surgical elective. It was amazing what I saw there. When I was in Latin America, I had thought, "How could poverty be any worse?" But my first night in Africa was like walking into a *National Geographic* magazine. There were pigs in the road. People used kerosene lamps because they had no electricity. You could smell all the spices from people cooking in their huts, but mixed with these exotic odors was the smell of urine. I was so distressed that I asked God, "Why are people living like this, when I live like I do in the U.S.?"

In Ghana we had some really serious fibroid tumor cases. One patient who arrived by taxi looked like she was nine months pregnant because of her fibroids. She needed surgery but wouldn't have survived because her hemoglobin was too low. They had no blood bank in Ghana, but the taxi driver who brought her to the hospital and her cousin both had compatible blood (O negative) and donated so we could operate.

But during the surgery, the patient started decompensating because of blood loss. The anesthesiologist told us, "All her vital signs are down. She's not going to make it. She needs more blood." "Well," I said, "I'm O negative too." So we did a transfusion directly from me to her on the spot. She survived the surgery. When she woke up afterwards and found out she had a white person's blood, she asked me, "Why did you give your life to me?" In Ghana they call blood "life." I told her, "Jesus gave His life for us so we could live." She was a Christian too. She hugged me and started praying to God and thanking Jesus. Later her daughter asked me, "Are we sisters now?" It was so sweet.

One common health problem for women in many parts of Africa is vaginal fistulas. I'd studied the topic in med school during my sub-internship in obstetrics and gynecology. In much of Africa it's actually a pediatric problem, because it occurs most often in young girls. Girls as young as 11 or 12 years old are sometimes forced to get married and they become pregnant, but their bodies are not fully grown and ready to deliver a baby. During labor the baby's head is too big for the immature birth canal and gets stuck. Because modern obstetrical care is often unavailable, labor goes on for days and the prolonged pressure of the baby's head on the wall of the vagina causes a hole or fistula into the bladder or rectum. If the fistula is into the bladder, the girl will constantly leak urine, if into the rectum, she will leak feces. A fistula needs surgical repair. It's not going to heal on its own.

While I was at Loma Linda, I went to Ethiopia on a mission elective with Hands of Mercy and E3 Partners. While I was there,

I found out that there was a fistula hospital in a nearby village. I went over and spoke with the doctor in charge and he invited me to the operating room to scrub in and see him perform a fistula repair. I spent two weeks volunteering in the fistula hospital. It was amazing to see how one surgery could change someone's life so much.

I would go early in the morning, before the hospital opened, and sit with the girls on the ground outside. I would find a dry spot among the puddles of urine, and I would smile at the girls and touch them. I didn't speak their language; they were from many different regions and spoke different languages. But I felt God wanted me to be with them and sit with them. Women who have this problem feel so ashamed; they feel cursed by God. They wear rags and spend most of their time outside because they leak urine. Nobody wants to be near them. Most of the girls lose the babies they have carried. Usually their husbands abandon them, and their parents don't want them back because they are such a burden and their problem is considered so shameful.

I grew to love these girls. I could see how human touch and compassion meant so much to them. The first few days, they just looked down at the ground. But after I spent every day with them for two weeks, they began to smile and wave at me when I came back. They loved to touch my hair. They wanted to braid it. They'd braid a section, then I'd have to go assist in surgery, and when I returned, they would braid a little more. It took a couple of days to finish.

I prayed, "God, I want to work with these fistula girls. I know I'm in pediatrics, but they're just kids! So if it's Your plan, someday help me connect with a fistula hospital." But I knew I didn't have the training or credentials to work there. You have to be an obstetrician/gynecologist or a urologic gynecologist to do that.

The following year, I went on a short-term mission trip to Sudan with Volunteers in Medical Missions supported by the Trinity Presbytery in South Carolina and then to Kenya with Genesis World Mission. Before I left, I attended a briefing about what to expect. They told us regarding Sudan, "You might die. The village is surrounded by land mines. You can only walk where the goats have gone—let them pave the way because if they haven't blown up, chances are you won't either. And there are tribes raiding cattle, and everyone's armed." I knew it was not the safest place in the world to go, yet it was where God was calling me, and that was the best place I could be. For me, that's always been my security: knowing I'm exactly where God wants me to be.

In Sudan I saw a patient named Sarah who was febrile and leaking urine. She was a young girl and she reeked. When I put the speculum in I could see pus and bits of tissue. The doctor I was working with confirmed my diagnosis—she was septic and had a fistula. Two weeks before, Sarah had been pregnant and had gone into labor and had walked day and night for three days to the hospital with her baby's head engaged in her pelvis. The baby was dead and Sarah had a complete detachment of the urethra and bladder. The doctors in the hospital removed the dead baby's body and sent Sarah home.

Now she was back at the hospital. The health officer told her there was nothing they could do for her. But I said, "No! There's a fistula hospital in Addis Ababa in Ethiopia, just across the river. I've been there." Well, he told me, "If it's across the river, she'll have to wait until the rainy season. And the motor on our only boat is broken, and the part won't be here for three months. And when the water is high enough she'll have to go upstream to cross because enemy tribesmen in this area would kill her. Once she crosses the river, there is no road for most of the trip to Addis Ababa so she'll need to use animals for transportation. Once everything is ready, it will probably take her three weeks to get to the hospital."

Here in the United States, we go to the emergency room and get antibiotics that day and have surgery the next. It's not like that in Sudan.

"But it's a hospital for women with this problem," I said. "She doesn't have to die!"

"Are you going to take on this project?" he asked me. "Because it's also going to cost a lot of money."

I answered, "Let me pray about it and I'll let you know." Then I looked in Sarah's eyes, heard her sigh, and saw a puddle of urine flow out of her. I thought, "God, I have to help her. You showed me the fistula hospital; You gave me that project in med school. I asked You to help me find a way to help these women, and here it is in Sudan, right in front of me."

So I told the health official I would be responsible. I told Sarah I was a Catholic physician and that I would pray for her healing. I also told her my plan: I hoped to coordinate my vacation from residency with the window of opportunity she had to get to

Ethiopia. I'd meet her and drive with her the last part of the journey
to the fistula hospital in Addis Ababa and back again. Sarah was fortunate because her husband loved her and had stayed with her.
They were both optimistic about my plan.

At that point I had to leave Sarah and Sudan and begin work
in Kenya. One day at lunch in the village in Kenya, my nurse said,
"Dr. Lori, you seem sad." I told her I was thinking about my
patient back in Sudan, and I told her Sarah's story. She said, "Why
can't Kenya help you? The African Inland Mission pilots travel
through Sudan on their flights," she said. "They could bring her
here to Kijabe Hospital."

I was worried about the cost, because Kenya is more
upscale than Ethiopia, and the fistula hospital in Ethiopia is free.
My nurse said, "Let's find out tonight. Kijabe is just a few miles
from here." We took a motorcycle, walked for miles, boarded a
taxi, and walked some more. That trip of a "few miles" took us
seven hours. At Kijabe Hospital we met Dr. Smith, an ob/gyn
with World Medical Mission. She had been trained in fistula
surgery and had a lot of experience repairing fistulas. She said,
"I'd love to do Sarah's surgery."

At that point my mission trip was over and I had to return to
residency at Loma Linda. When I got back to California I emailed
Africa Inland Mission and made contact with the pilot. Sight
unseen the pilot told me he would love to help. God's hand was
truly at work as I organized all of this with people I did not know
from thousands of miles away in the United States.

When the pilot airlifted Sarah out of Sudan for her surgery,
another woman came with her. That was the result of a meeting I'd
had previously with the village commissioner in Sudan, asking permission to take Sarah out of the country for surgery. He had asked
me, "Why just Sarah? There are many other women with this
problem in their huts. We know they are there because we smell
them. They don't come out because it's so shameful."

The commissioner asked if we would try to help other women
in Sarah's village. I agreed and after I left for Kenya, he went
through the streets with a loudspeaker to announce that treatment
for this problem was available. That's how Miriam came forward.
She had suffered with a fistula for 20 years. When it started, she
went from wearing beautiful traditional Sudanese clothing to
wearing rags and smelling bad all the time. For 20 years, no one
touched her or bothered with her. She lived a life of loneliness and

isolation. But she had so much faith that she spent her time sewing a beautiful new dress and praying that someday she could take off her smelly rags and wear it.

So when Miriam heard the commissioner on the loudspeaker and heard from others in the village that Sarah was going for surgery, she came forward. It was verified that she had a fistula, and she flew out with Sarah for Dr. Smith to attempt the repair. Miriam brought with her a bag containing her beautiful dress. The surgery for both women was successful. When Miriam was told she was cured, she put on her beautiful dress in the hospital ward and started dancing and singing praises to God, telling of how God had healed her. Like the hemorrhaging woman in the Gospel, she had been healed by her faith. She boarded the plane back to Sudan in her beautiful dress, with her rags in the bag.

This past year two other Sudanese girls with fistulas turned up in Sarah and Miriam's village, and we were able to arrange to airlift them out all through email communications. It cost about $1,000 for each girl to get the surgery, mostly to pay for transportation, visas and food costs, since Kijabe Hospital doesn't charge anything. We did no fundraising; the money has just happened. It's been amazing how people have come forward to make it possible for me to do all this work. My church in California, St. Joseph the Worker in Loma Linda, has supported much of my mission work. There's a semi-retired physician and professor of radiation sciences who has donated to each of my trips. He tells me, "Lori, I can't go but you can."

I was at Loma Linda reading an email about these two additional girls and how they needed the fistula surgery, but it was uncertain when the money would be available for them. My attending physician saw me checking my emails and asked me why I was smiling. I said, "Oh, Dr. Cutler, it's an amazing story." I told him about these fistula girls and their problems. Since this was my nephrology rotation, I mentioned that many of these girls die of bacterial kidney infections.

Some time later that day, Dr. Cutler told me to check my mailbox. In it was a large check. A nurse who had also heard the story gave another $300. I didn't even know she was listening! Several others donated and in the space of one day, God provided everything we needed, just through sharing that story.

This fistula project is dear to my heart, because I had started reading about the fistulas in medical school and thinking how tragic they were. I can't imagine leaking urine all the time and not being touched or loved or cared for. God brought me to Ethiopia to see the hospital, and then to Sudan to help the girls there. I'm excited to go back to Sudan this spring. I've been praying that another fistula girl would show up that we could help. Perhaps God wants me someday to form an organization to help the fistula girls, but I will leave that up to Him. I just need to see where God leads with this.

There are so many frustrating obstacles to practicing medicine in Africa. On our last day in Ethiopia, we saw a child, a 10-year-old girl named Aisha, who had a brain tumor. Because she staggered when she walked, she was bumping into the walls of her hut. Most of the time her mother carried her so that she wouldn't hurt herself. The family was very poor. They had been told nothing could be done for their daughter. "Can you do anything, please?" her mother asked us.

We'd seen so many neurologically devastated kids in the mission clinic, kids we could treat for seizures but not cure. But something about Aisha made us all think she might have a benign and treatable brain tumor. We thought, "How hard is it to get a CT scan?" Well, we didn't realize how hard it was. We were told she would have to travel three days by bus from her village in the Sudan to Addis Ababa in Ethiopia. We all prayed about this and felt God was calling us to help Aisha. We raised the $300 for the CT scan and for the bus ride with her family accompanying her. I was scheduled to spend a month in Ethiopia and was able to stay with Aisha and her mother throughout the process.

When Aisha got to the Christian mission hospital in Addis, they did the scan and found a huge mass. A missionary neurosurgeon agreed to operate. He was the son and grandson of missionaries, and was training Ethiopian doctors to do neurosurgery. Aisha had surgery in December, the tumor was malignant, but the surgical resection went well and she had a smooth recovery.

When I left Aisha and her mother, I was in tears. She asked her mother, "Why is the doctor crying?" I told her through the translator that they were tears of joy, because I was so thankful to have been part of God's plan to help her, that God could use us to touch her life. Several months later I saw how much Aisha had improved when I went to visit them. Aisha ran out of her hut to greet me. I would never have known that this was the same little girl who once had been walking into walls.

But a few months later, I got word that Aisha had what sounded like meningitis. I got a call from the hospital in Ethiopia, the staff had heard from the village that Aisha was having seizures and was comatose. They thought it was either meningitis or a brain abscess. She needed high dose IV antibiotics. The doctor in her village had seen her, but all he had available was one shot of antibiotics and some oral doses. A short time later I got the news that Aisha died of the infection.

During my next trip to Ethiopia a few months after Aisha's death, I talked to the village doctor. He told me, "This is what happens. This is why in the beginning we told her there was nothing we could do for her. When these kids have surgery, a lot of them die later anyway, from infections and complications we can't take care of." In third world countries, the hospital may or may not be stocked with antibiotics. It may or may not have a chest tube. It may or may not have oxygen. That's just the reality in a small village in Ethiopia.

I also went to visit Aisha's mom. She had sold her family's goats to pay for Aisha's care, even though we had done everything we could to help out financially. It was a very tearful visit. It was hard for me not to see Aisha running out of the family's hut with all her brothers and sisters. But even so, her mom told me, "Through this I saw how much God loved Aisha, that He sent these white people to care for her in her last months. I feel our family has grown. You and the others who tried to help are part of her life, part of my family. I'm okay with her going."

I was glad to be part of her life too. I remember after Aisha's surgery, people were asking her mother in the clinic, "Who is that white person with your daughter?" She told them, "This doctor loves Aisha and helped her get surgery to heal her." Then the other waiting patients wanted to touch me, thinking I had some healing power. But Aisha's mom told them, "No, no! All these doctors say the glory goes to God. God is the healer." It made me think of the stories from the Bible of the good news of Jesus spreading by word of mouth. That's exactly what Aisha's mom was doing. I prayed, "God, Your name is still being praised through this little girl's life."

I had another patient in Sudan named Nasor, a two-year old, with a Wilms' tumor.[5] His mom came to us on her way to throw him into the river. His abdomen was very swollen and the village doctors had given him worm medication, thinking that was the problem, but it hadn't helped. Then they realized that the swelling

---

5. A Wilms' tumor is a malignant cancer of the kidney that occurs in children.

was due to a huge abdominal mass and told the mom that they couldn't do surgery or offer any other help to the child.

The father had kicked them out of the house and told the mother to get rid of Nasor because he was a burden on the family. Nasor needed all of the mom's attention and that kept her from her duties as the youngest wife in the hut. Nasor's mom had walked for days to reach the village where she had been raised. She was going to throw Nasor in the river, but she wanted to see her own mother first. On her way she noticed the medical clinic and decided to bring him to us.

We examined Nasor and realized he must have a Wilms' tumor. These tumors have a good cure rate, so we made arrangements to have him airlifted out to Kijabe Hospital. He had a surgical resection by a missionary surgeon, who said that the tumor was contained within the kidney and showed good histology. Nasor's projected five-year survival was 92 percent. But to complete his treatment he needed chemotherapy, and in Kenya there aren't a lot of chemotherapy drugs available. One of the drugs Nasor needed was actinomycin-D, which is very expensive—at least $500 a vial. And Nasor would need several vials.

One of the doctors at Kijabe was from Germany and said he would write to contacts in Germany to see what could be done. When I went back to the United States, I called some oncologists and pharmacists I knew and asked if they could help me get some actinomycin-D. They all told me it would cost thousands of dollars. I prayed, "Lord, Nasor has had his surgery. I know You will make a way when there seems to be no way." And sure enough, He did.

Finally, I called Lundbeck, the pharmaceutical company that makes actinomycin-D. I spoke with a woman at the company and told her the story of little Nasor. Within 24 hours emails went to the company's branches all over Europe asking them to see if there were vials of repackaged drug that were unsellable but could still be used.

Just before Nasor was due to start his chemotherapy, we got word that Lundbeck was donating all the actinomycin-D that he needed. In fact, the company donated so many vials that three other children with Wilms' tumors were also treated. Nasor's chemo went well, and now he's waiting to go back home to Sudan.

On the last day of chemotherapy, pictures were taken of Nasor for the pharmaceutical company's newsletter, so that all the company's employees could read his story and see the difference they had made in his life. I saw the picture of Nasor's mom kissing him and saying, "I'm so glad I didn't throw you away, Nasor." Before this chapter in her life, she had never wanted anything to do with God but now she said, "There has to be a God, and God has to have loved Nasor."

Last summer I finished my residency at Loma Linda. I was at the airport, walking from the terminal to the parking garage, when a car hit me. The driver was a young kid texting on his cell phone. When he looked up, it was too late. He swerved to try to avoid me, but he ran over my foot and the impact threw me to the ground. Anyhow, that's what the witness said. I was knocked out, so I don't remember what happened. When I woke up I found out I had a broken fibula and tibia of my left leg. The fractures had to be surgically repaired with a bone graft, plates and screws. I'll need a second surgery in a year, hopefully just to have the hardware removed.

I just didn't understand it. Here I was, finished with my residency and ready to go to work full time, either here in this country or in the mission field. But now I was stuck in bed for two months, and I didn't know whether I'd ever walk again. I also had a brachial plexus injury, so I couldn't use my arm, not even with a crutch. I wondered if I would be able to practice medicine again. How would I hold babies? How would I hold an otoscope to look in kids' ears?

"God," I prayed, "I've served You in the mission field all this time. If I never walk again, how am I going to go back to Sudan? What is this accident for? I don't get this. I'm a doctor. I don't want to be a patient. How am I supposed to see You in this?" But God found a way to use this setback to my benefit. Through this suffering as I searched for meaning, I really grew closer to God. I thought, "Lori, you're always telling your patients to have faith and trust in God. Now *you're* having a hard time." I thought of all my patients and remembered that everyone suffers. Through my questioning, I grew closer to understanding Jesus' suffering. We don't like it, but it's part of our existence. I learned that we all have to suffer in some way.

Before the accident, I thought of myself as a compassionate person. But if anything, I am so much more sensitive now to children with disabilities. I thought I understood why the parents of children with cerebral palsy were late to appointments. But now I *really* understand how things take longer when you're dealing with a disability. It's a totally different understanding of suffering and how we can unite our struggles with Christ's struggle.

Now, instead of getting upset with God, we can just say, "Okay, God I don't understand this. You show me and give me joy in this." And God will meet that need. He helped me to see my suffering as something that is shaping me, helping to deepen my faith. I prayed, "God, if You let me walk again, these feet will go wherever You want me to go. These hands will serve You no matter what."

My orthopedic surgeon, Dr. Yu, was a Christian. He used to pray with me, and I loved being the recipient of his prayers. I was awake during my surgery, and Dr. Yu told me my posterior tibial tendon was ruptured. He said, "I might have to dig a little bit for it. Pray that I find it. Start praying, Lori!" And I prayed.

This doctor, who is such a great surgeon, is also a man of God. He was not thinking, "I'm going to find this tendon with my surgical skill." He was thinking of God and asking, "Please help, Lord." It mattered to me that at every follow-up appointment, he prayed before he did anything else. For example, he prayed before my x-ray to see if my bone was healing. That's the kind of doctor I want to be.

After surgery I had to go to physical therapy. I saw suffering there too, when I was still seeking to understand it myself. I met several young kids who had been in car accidents. One kid had been trying out for the wrestling team when another wrestler came down on him and fractured one of his vertebrae. Now he can't walk. Another kid told me that since he was paralyzed, his parents were overwhelmed and started blaming each other. They are now divorced and his life is a mess. When I began physical therapy, I knew I would probably walk again, but here were these kids who might never be able to.

I prayed, "God, if I'm having a hard time understanding You, what must it be like for them? Here I am sharing the whirlpool with them but I also want to talk to them. My heart is sad for them. But if I want to talk to them about You, how can I make them see what an awesome God You are? I want to encourage them to find their strength in You, as I have. What do I say?" And sure enough, before I could say much, one of them asked me, "If there is a God, why doesn't He make these neurons come back so I can walk?"

I couldn't come up with a satisfactory answer for that.

Shortly afterwards, I heard of the Catholic Medical Association's conference on "The Theology of Suffering." I knew it was exactly what I needed. So I went to the conference, and through the lectures and time spent in Eucharistic adoration and prayer, I began to feel God speaking to me, "I am with you in the suffering. It all has a purpose." Through the conference, I realized that helping others who are suffering, like the kids I met in physical therapy, might involve more than words or actions. Sometimes helping others means just listening to them and letting them know you'll pray for them, so that God will reveal Himself to them. He is there for them in their suffering. That we can be sure of.

So as it turned out, my accident was a gift in disguise. Without it, I would never have met those injured children or had the opportunity to pray for them, as I still do. I would never have attended the CMA conference if the accident hadn't happened. Through this, God has brought people into my life who have encouraged me, as a physician and as a person. So I can rejoice in this, because it really has taught me a lot.

To feed my spiritual life, I read the Bible and spend time in prayer daily. I go to Mass and to Eucharistic adoration. Since my parents do adoration every day, when I'm home, I go with them. I grew up doing that and I love spending time with the Lord. I pray a lot and I share fellowship with other Christians, which is very encouraging for me because it allows me to see how God works in other people's lives. A lot of my friends are Christians and physicians, and they tell stories of miracles they've seen: "How else could this patient have been healed except by God?" These kinds of stories really make you grow in your faith.

I also read books for spiritual nourishment. Right now I'm reading *Making Sense Out of Suffering*, a wonderful book by Peter Kreeft, a Catholic writer. I'm also about to read John Paul II's *On the Christian Meaning of Human Suffering*.

I used to think that the mission field was in far away places, but I've come to see that it's wherever I am. There are people in need everywhere, people who need to hear about God. I just keep praying, "Okay, God, where are You calling me for the next period of my life?" Then I go wherever that is. By doing this I find such joy and I discover that God will use me in ways I could never have imagined.

Once I finished my residency training, I began looking around for a regular job. I found a job in California and start soon.

I'll be doing outpatient and inpatient pediatrics and have a month off every year for missions. When I was a resident, I always had an attending physician to help me out. Now I'm becoming an attending and it's a little scary, kind of like "the buck stops here." But Loma Linda gave me a good education and I know God is going to be with me. I'm really excited to be finished with my training and able to start work. I love being a doctor. When I was in bed for two months after the accident, I would open the window just so I could hear the kids playing on the nearby school playground. And I would pray, "Oh, God, someday I'll be a doctor with them again. Someday I will. Someday I will."

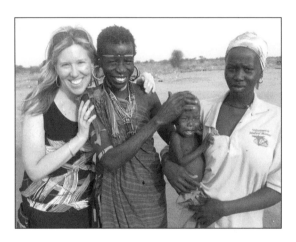

Dr. Lori Warzecki with little Nasor,
his mother and grandmother in Sudan.

— *Ad Majorem Dei Gloriam* —

2

Dr. Timothy Flanigan

THE GREAT INVITATION

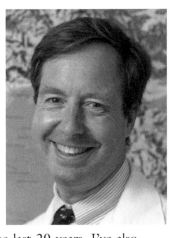

I'm an infectious disease doctor, specializing in treating HIV/AIDS. I provide clinical care and direct clinical research, integrated with teaching at the Brown University Medical School. For the last 20 years, I've also run a half-day clinic at the Rhode Island State Prison for patients with HIV, which I really enjoy.

I'm also Roman Catholic. I'm an "Irish twin"; my sister Sheila (who's a nun) and I were born less than a year apart. And I'm currently in the process of considering a vocation to the diaconate. The Faith is such a beautiful gift and I feel incredibly lucky to be Catholic.

Although I'm a cradle Catholic, my faith was invigorated when I was an undergraduate at Dartmouth. A typical New England college, Dartmouth had a very secular environment. But we had a close Catholic community that gathered at Aquinas House, a student center run by a wonderful Catholic priest named Father Bill Nolan. He was a great priest who loved sharing the Sacraments and talking about God's goodness and grace. In fact, a number of students chose vocations to the priesthood and religious life thanks to his influence.

At Dartmouth, I began to realize what a gift the Faith is, and began to accept it as my own. We spent time reading G. K. Chesterton, C. S. Lewis, J. R. R. Tolkien, and Charles Williams and thinking and talking about the great adventure of life—to risk, to dare, to fail, to be invited to explore the meaning of our existence, whether through love, pain, suffering or mercy. College is a great time to delve into the most important questions with which we all grapple. It's a time when you're trying to figure out "why are we here?" Your parents aren't around anymore and it's just as easy to get totally drunk as it is to take a hike or to pray for an hour and nobody is around who cares which of these three you choose.

College also is a time when you deal with pain and sorrow, excitement and disappointment, success and failure. Whether it's being rejected by a girl you like, or reading a great book, or going overseas and traveling in another country, you're exploring your part in the great adventure. In college you begin to realize what people are truly like, with all their warts and all their issues. It's a time when, in small ways, you can begin to see what being alive really means, what the bigger picture is.

What stuck with me is that we're all invited to this great adventure of life and we're all accepting that invitation to greater or lesser degrees every day. That's scary, but it's also invigorating to realize that it matters how we respond to the invitation. It matters because God, his Son, Jesus Christ, and his Mother, Mary, really care about us.

College campuses breed skepticism, relativism and secularism. The prevailing attitude is: There is no "truth;" there is no invitation. You should do whatever it takes to feel good and the more pleasure, the better. That kind of environment makes it pretty easy to fall into *ennui*, despair and boredom, because nothing seems truly important.

After a while many college students realize that this mindset is a dead end. A life measured by fun and pleasure is not an adventure and is, in fact, quite meaningless. In the long run, it doesn't really matter if you have a good croissant or a regular old muffin, whether your coffee is from Starbucks or Dunkin Donuts. What does matter is the fact that someone out there is starving for food, for love, or both. There are big issues out there, and you're asked to play a role. Your life has meaning. You count. You're invited to be "part of the Great Adventure."

C. S. Lewis spoke about life as a great play. We're all personally invited by our Lord to play a role on the stage in this great drama. Our role matters. We don't know how important our role is and we don't need to know ahead of time. When we first step out on that stage, we think it's *our* play; that it's all about *us*. We have to be taught through life's lessons that it's not *our* play—it's *His* play. We're not asked to be the star; we're just asked to play our specific role, even if it is difficult, and it usually is, and even if it's not the role we think we should play.

You can find an example of this idea in J. R. R. Tolkien's

Lord of the Rings. In that story, each person matters, whether hobbit, elf, or dwarf. A casual reader might think that the wizard Gandalf is the most important character. Well, he's certainly the most powerful, but he's not the most important. Although Sam, Frodo, Merry and Pippin appear to be insignificant hobbits from Middle Earth, their roles in the battle against evil make them the most important characters.

It takes a long time to figure this out. As we are learning our roles, we're going to step on toes and misspeak our lines, stumble and fall, say the wrong things. The important thing is that we're willing to accept the invitation and try. And if we flub it, will we keep going? We're asked to keep trying. For me, as for a lot of people, college was the first place where I began to ponder these exhilarating ideas.

In college I didn't really have much of an idea about what I wanted to do with my life. I was a history major but I also took pre-med courses. My senior thesis, not a literary masterpiece by any stretch, was titled "Light from the Dark Ages: Thomism in the 20th Century." It was mostly a compilation of quotes from The *Dumb Ox*, G. K. Chesterton's book on St. Thomas Aquinas, with some Jacques Maritain and a few others thrown in.

I spent a semester working in a bank, and although it was interesting, I didn't find it very exciting. Then I went up to the northernmost tip of Newfoundland with the Quebec Labrador Foundation, where I volunteered as an orderly in a hospital in the town of St. Anthony. My job was to wheel patients here and there and to follow the doctors around. It may not sound like much, but I thought, "Wow, *this* is really exciting."

That excitement led me to Cornell Medical School in 1979 after graduating from Dartmouth. I have continued to be fascinated by medicine. I'm not alone—just look at how many people watch the TV show *House.* One of the things I love about medicine is that you're always interacting intimately with human nature and you find out about how people respond to illness, imperfection, and suffering. One day you're caring for a middle-aged man who has lost his leg due to severe diabetes; the next day you're helping a family deal with their father who has just had a heart attack; then you're treating a young woman with a life-threatening abscess. In medicine you're constantly rubbing shoulder to shoulder with humanity, giving you an intimate view of the extraordinary drama of life.

Of course, we also see patients who are angry, frustrated, or fearful. We see patients who don't rise up to the challenge, who are not heroic, who are bitter and resentful. But change is always possible. That fear can turn to hope and the anger to forgiveness. The interaction between doctor and patient is very intimate. You're not going to engage at that level with your accountant. But with your doctor, you frequently do interact in a deeply personal way. A doctor can ask all kinds of questions that no one in other professions would consider asking. This role is an amazing honor and privilege that one has to respect; that intimacy is very special.

After Cornell I did my internship at the University of Pennsylvania, where I met my future wife, Luba, on our orientation day. We started going out together and our relationship continued through our residencies. Two-thirds of the way through residency, Luba decided that she was going to do a fellowship in hematology and oncology at Case Western Reserve University in Ohio and I thought I'd better do a fellowship there as well if I didn't want to lose her. I chose infectious disease as my specialty because tropical diseases sounded interesting.

That was in the early 1980s when the AIDS epidemic was upon us in full force. At that time we were calling it GRID— gay-related immunodeficiency. We were caring for young men who were sick with a devastating illness that caused terrible pain and stripped away their dignity. Their symptoms included awful rashes, diarrhea, weight loss and nausea, and they were faced with the stigma of being HIV positive. They didn't feel good about their bodies; they felt dirty and "infected."

Particularly in those early days when we didn't know much about how the disease spread, a lot of people didn't want to touch patients with HIV. Even health care providers would say, "Oh, yes, I'll take care of them, but I'd rather not touch them." Always there was the unspoken question: Could I get it from them? Patients with HIV were the "new lepers."

I took care of my first AIDS patient in 1983 on my second night on call as an intern. I was actually told I didn't have to take care of *this* patient because he had this mysterious disease. But when asked by my senior resident, I responded, "Sure, I'd be happy to help take care of him." So we gowned and we gloved and we put on masks.

Brian (not his real name) was a young man in his 30s who had severe AIDS. He had lost a tremendous amount of weight and he had pneumonia. For the next three weeks, I took care of him. He got a little better, went home, but relapsed and came back into the hospital. Every day I went in to draw his blood, examine him and talk about his illness and his treatment.

Taking care of Brian was very moving for me. Here was a gay man who had been raised as a Catholic but obviously had been alienated from the Church. Yet Brian prayed the rosary every day. *Every day.* I'd walk by his room and see him with his rosary beads. I was awed by his relationship with Jesus and Mary because it was so real and so deep. It was truly extraordinary to see how he had reconciled with the Church and how deeply his faith had grown. It wasn't just a question of the difficulty of being gay and being Catholic. Brian knew he was terribly ill and he was scared and in pain. Yet he knew the Lord loved him and accepted him, and in his need he returned to God. The Lord's invitation to us transcends a lot of our difficulties. We may have stumbling blocks but God reaches over them with his grace, mercy, and love—with his invitation. It's easy for us to think that the invitation is only there for people like *us*, but not there for people like *that*. But that view is wrong.

Brian's mother was constantly with him. They had a very loving relationship, which was a privilege to see. In medicine one sees the kind of heroism that illness calls forth from patients, their family members, and others who work with them. Every day I drew his blood. This was painful for him because he didn't have good veins and I was an intern with little experience. Sometimes I had to stick him three, four, and five times. He and his mother never complained. That was real heroism. But it was quiet. There were no trumpets, no banners; it was not written up anywhere. Day in and day out, until Brian died, I had the privilege of witnessing that heroism.

As the AIDS epidemic was galloping along, I became determined to step in and see if I could make a difference as an infectious disease doctor. There happened to be a parasitic infection associated with AIDS called cryptosporidiosis.[6] Nobody knew how to treat it; there were no effective antibiotics. I thought, "Gosh, this would be worthwhile to do research on. If we found something that worked, we'd be able to help a lot of people." For many years, I worked on that project while taking

---

6. Cryptosporidiosis is a parasitic infection of the intestines that causes diarrhea. In most patients the symptoms are mild, but in those with AIDS it can be severe and fatal.

care of patients. Ironically, it was effective treatment for the underlying HIV that cured AIDS-related cryptosporidiosis.

I consider myself lucky to have been able to see the evolution of effective treatment for HIV/AIDS. There are so many diseases for which we still don't have effective treatments: lung cancer, cirrhosis of the liver, emphysema, to name just a few. But during my professional lifetime, I've witnessed HIV/AIDS treatment evolve from nothing, to poor, to moderate, to highly successful treatment. These days, for many patients, the treatment is as simple as one pill a day, which can drive HIV viral replication to non-detectable levels. We can put AIDS into total remission and patients can recover 100 percent from HIV immunodeficiency. The patient still has the HIV infection, but we can reverse the immune destruction that has occurred. So I tell my HIV patients that if they take care of themselves, there's no reason that they can't live to be 70, 80, or even 90 years old.

The most important thing is that they must be willing to be engaged in their own care. Are they willing to take their medicines? If they smoke, are they willing to stop smoking? If they use drugs, are they willing to stop using them? If they have other illnesses such as diabetes or hypertension, are they willing to engage in treatment? With that kind of involvement, our treatment of the patient with HIV can be extraordinarily effective. It's really amazing to have seen such a change in my lifetime and to know that I've participated in a small way.

Our clinical research also has been fulfilling. We challenge ourselves to give better care to HIV patients who are substance users and to find ways to provide family-centered HIV care. I'm involved in international projects where we ask ourselves how we can provide HIV care in countries that have fewer resources than the United States. Working in Africa, we try to figure out how we can provide generic medications made in India that are super cheap and work very well, and then work on teaching people how to use them. Further, my work in prisons here has made me concerned about the spread of HIV and tuberculosis in the prisons in Ukraine and elsewhere in Eastern Europe.

In the early days of the AIDS epidemic when we had no treatment, I spent time visiting dying patients in their homes. It's a privilege to take care of patients at the end of their lives when home visits are so important. The act of dying is painful, scary, and yet phenomenally meaningful. Those of us in the medical profession often can't change the course of an illness, but we can be the guides for our patients along the way.

Our role is similar to that of a guide on a hike into the wilderness. Patients don't know what's around the next corner or what the path is like up that mountain. So they need a guide. They still have to walk that trail, but it helps to know if the trail ahead will be bumpy or rough, steep or scary, with precipices on each side. In medicine we can't always change the path, but sometimes we can make the path easier to follow by literally and figuratively holding the patient's hand.

When a patient is dying, you as a doctor know what to expect, and you need to be honest. If a patient is stable and says, "Doctor, am I going to die?" you might respond, "Well, I think for now you're doing okay. If you want to plan to try to get out and do something, go for it!" Or, if somebody is *really* dying, you might want to say to the family members, "You'd better get everybody here, because I think your loved one isn't going to be with us for more than another day or two." And you always add, "I really don't know, and I hope I'm wrong," because doctors are frequently proven wrong. When that happens, it's wonderful.

At the end of life, being at home is almost always preferable to being in the hospital where an inherent dehumanization takes place, which you have to accept to a certain degree. This is especially true about hospital intensive care. Being in an ICU and being intubated is awful. When you're on a ventilator, a breathing machine, you can't talk and half the time you're naked. Your dignity is thrown out the window. Now, there's nothing wrong with intensive-care-unit medicine. When you need it, you want it to be there; but if you're dying and it's not going to help, you shouldn't be there. You should be at home with hospice care, with your family and friends surrounded by their care and comfort.

In my experience, American society does not know how to deal with suffering. In India and in Africa, where there is tremendous physical and emotional suffering, people accept it. It's like the rain; it just happens. We're supposed to be there to comfort each other through suffering, but we can't avoid it. That attitude is uncommon in America. Suffering is not "supposed to happen"— yet it does. And why? Why does one child get sick and die of influenza but another gets better and survives? We don't know. We don't understand it. The pain and suffering are so intense that we begin to question how God can let it happen.

All we know is that Jesus Christ suffered terribly at the Passion and on the Cross, and He did it out of love for us. His suffering is filled with tremendous meaning and grace, and in some way is tied to salvation, to the forgiveness of our sins. Our Christian faith tells us Jesus is with us in our pain and suffering.

Every Lent, we show the film *The Passion of the Christ* to the guys in the high-security prison here. It resonates pretty powerfully with them. Jesus was a prisoner, and they are in prison. He was treated really badly and sometimes they are treated pretty badly. Any pain the inmates feel, He has felt worse. Jesus has been rejected, alienated, tortured and abandoned. Yet He willingly endured all that for us.

Often in our sickness we feel pain and abandonment. Our comfort is that He is here with us, holding our hands while we are suffering. Don't ever think you can "explain" someone's suffering to them. You can't ever say you know how they feel, because you don't. You shouldn't ever say, "There must be some good that will come out of it," because that makes people feel worse. However, you can say, "Jesus is there with you. He will help you." He's there with us, even though we may not acknowledge Him or choose to look at Him. A lot of times we don't, but He's still there. That's why the Crucifix is so powerful.

When I was a doctor in training, treating HIV patients was a great challenge. Now I'd say that one of the greatest challenges in American medicine is drug addiction. Alcohol, heroin, cocaine—drug addiction just poisons the body, mind, and soul. Addiction is so destructive, so awful. People who are using often do terrible things and have terrible things done to them. How can we better care for patients with drug addictions? It's a whole new frontier, one worth delving into and figuring out how to do with love and compassion.

The heroin addict, the cocaine user, and the alcoholic all suffer terribly. But sometimes only when you hit "rock bottom," do you begin to understand good and evil, mercy and repentance, love and acceptance. The same is often true for those in prison; they also have hit bottom and are more open to God's grace and goodness. In some ways, the message of God's mercy is easier to communicate to people who are in prison because they have learned a little humility. Believe me, if you're incarcerated, you're humble. Where there is great suffering, there can be great grace.

I've been privileged to know patients who have managed to

completely transform their lives. For over 10 years, for example, I have taken care of a woman who was in jail, had been a crack user and was a heroin addict. But finally after 20 years of addiction, she embraced Narcotics Anonymous, and with help and support from her family and a lot of prayer, she's clean now and she's been doing great for over five years. Her worries today are the same as anyone else's: Is it going to snow? How can I control my diabetes? What's going on with my family? She has a great sense of humor and is very grateful that she has been able to stay sober every day. It's a beautiful thing to witness.

Often when people change, they do it quietly, without fanfare. They might be challenged, but through grace they are able to stay sober, every day. And they're quiet about it. They're just grateful. That's the extraordinary part of this great dance, this adventure of life. We only see a little of it, yet it's going on around us all the time.

Why don't we see it? Maybe we are taught to see through secular lenses. Our society does not so much deny religious truth and the love of God, the Father and his Son, as it ignores them. Society doesn't say, "God does not exist." Instead it says, "Let's worry about our new car and all our text messages. Let's worry about taking a nice vacation down in the Caribbean. Let's worry about whether other people admire us. Let's think about these things. You can always think later about 'the invitation' and life's deeper meaning. Let's turn the volume up so high that we don't need to listen to what the Lord is asking of us." The world is not so much railing against God as ignoring Him, and ultimately that leads to hopelessness and despair.

Instead we should be saying, "Holy cow! The Lord is inviting us to follow Him. That's much more important than everything else we're doing. So time-out!"

We all need a time-out every now and then to think about life's deeper meaning. As HIV treatments have gotten better and I've gotten older, I've thought about studying to be a deacon. I don't have a good explanation of how I felt called, but I can make an observation: The institutional Catholic Church is often marginalized, particularly here in North America. In recent years it has shrunk financially, and we've had the terrible sexual scandals that have undermined its credibility and trustworthiness. The Church has been pushed aside as society has become more secularized, whether by Hollywood, the media, or academia. Other respected voices shun it. It's not considered cool. Jesus' invitation to life, forgiveness and grace is not heard as much as it was in earlier times.

You mention Communion or Confession and many respond, "What, you mean that silly, superstitious practice of Catholics?" Or maybe they were raised Catholic, but they haven't thought of that in 30 years and they might harbor anger and resentment against the Church. Yet God can transcend these difficulties. God still speaks in many ways, and one way is through the institutional Church. It would be wonderful if I could play a role. Hopefully by being a deacon I can participate more fully in the work of God and of the Church.

In various ways, my faith has always played a role in my work as a physician. I once took care of a woman in her 30s with three young children. She had aggressive leukemia and it wasn't responding to chemotherapy. She had been a very devout Catholic, yet she told me, "I've stopped praying. I haven't talked to God for three years." She stopped because she didn't know how to pray. She didn't realize that she could be angry with God, that she could yell and scream at Him. She needed so desperately to know that He was there, but she didn't know how to talk to God. It seemed to her that God had given her this awful illness and He was taking her away from her three children.

I could understand how she felt, because I had always been taught to pray in church but not to swear, yell, scream, or cry in anger at Jesus. But people need to know that responding to God this way is okay, when that's how you feel. Jesus is there; He loves us and wants us to be honest. It's just like a moody kid. No parents likes it when their kid yells and screams. But I can tell you, as a parent, that it's a lot better to be yelled and screamed at by your kid than to have no communication at all. When your child runs away from home, there's nothing you want more than to have them back at home, even if it means your child is yelling and screaming in your face.

Prayer is about bringing our real needs and concerns to God. At 2:00 a.m. when I'm awake and worried, I pray to Mary for our children. I ask her to give them a hug and to watch over them. When I'm too anxious, the rosary really works well for me. I wonder whether sometimes we can't sleep because God wants us to turn to Him for help.

I find the most important things in my own spiritual life are the Sacraments. You go through a lot of highs and lows in life—

times when you feel very close to God, and other times when your relationship with Him seems more distant, more dry and disconnected. No matter how you're feeling, it's important to keep going to Confession and to Mass. It's easy when you're feeling inspired, but I think it's particularly crucial when you're not inspired, when you're tired and worn out. For me, going to Confession is like going to the dentist. I hate the thought of it and I don't want to do it ... but I feel so much better after I've gone. What an amazing thing it is to hear the priest say, "I absolve you from your sins in the name of the Father, and of the Son, and of the Holy Spirit." This isn't subtle stuff; this is a big gun. This is nuclear! Confession and absolution are offered to everyone, free of charge!

Prayer, the Sacraments, and faith are closely connected to healing and the alleviation of suffering. Seeing and participating in this connection is one of the great privileges of medical practice. We know that spiritual support can be helpful in facing illness. There's good scientific data to support this. Just look at the oncology literature: People who profess a spiritual faith have a better prognosis; they're happier and more hopeful. We know that faith is a good thing medically, and we should encourage and support it while being totally respectful of the diversity of beliefs. You do that by asking patients open-ended questions and following their lead.

So you can ask a patient, "Do you pray? Do you go to a church?" If the patient says "No, but I'd like to," you can suggest that he go around and look at different churches. You might ask, "How were you raised?" If the answer is "Well, I was raised a Roman Catholic," you can suggest that they visit several Catholic churches. Maybe they'll exclaim, "Oh, I couldn't stand church when I was growing up!" "Well," I would respond, "the Catholic Church is not the same today as it was 30 or 40 years ago. Go check it out—you might be surprised."

Some people might say, "I read the Bible, but I can't stand going to church." I tell them, "Great. You should keep reading the Bible. Maybe you ought to be doing that with some other people. Maybe you can find someone else who shares that interest." Half-jokingly, I always ask my patients, "Does it cost anything? No? Well, then, hey—check it out." I don't argue with patients or try to convince them. I give suggestions.

In my experience, nurses tend to have a very strong faith and they are generally more comfortable talking about it with patients than doctors are. I think too, that here in the Northeast we shy away from talking openly about matters of faith, but that's not as true in other parts of the country.

Occasionally, but not often, I pray with patients. If they're Christian, I use the Our Father, which I like because it cuts across and transcends denominational boundaries—that's a really nice thing. If a patient says he's Catholic and that's clearly important to him, I try to make sure a priest knows that he's in the hospital so he can come by for a pastoral visit. That can be such a good and important thing. It's amazing to me how often somebody is in the hospital doing poorly and nobody thinks to call the person's minister, priest or rabbi. Gosh, that's sad. It goes back to what I said before: Most people aren't atheists; they just ignore the presence of God. And that's wrong. Our job is to acknowledge that presence in a way that is considerate and respectful of the diversity of beliefs.

Brian, that first AIDS patient of mine, back in 1983, was a man who, according to the world's view, should have been alienated from God because he was gay. Yet his situation reveals how those extraordinary gifts of comfort, mercy and love in the Sacraments of the Catholic Church can transcend our preconceived notions. Just because someone is gay, like Brian, or a hardcore crack user who hasn't thought about going to church for 20 years, you may think that goodness and grace are closed to them, but you would be wrong. Anyone can ask for and receive grace in abundance. It doesn't mean that there isn't a huge challenge ahead for that person, a huge amount of sin and suffering to face up to—of course there is. But someone who's living in a crack house, having sex every night with a different person, using drugs, treating people terribly, can still return to God and be fully forgiven. Just look at the Prodigal Son.[7]

And of course the converse, unfortunately, is also true. People can close their hearts off to God's offer of love and redemption. It's scary and startling to think that you can be going to church, following all the rules, and doing everything you're supposed to do according to the world's view, and yet still reject God. That's startling to me. You've got to open up your heart to Him.

It's incredible what people go through in this drama of life. A patient of mine, who is on dialysis, has had both legs amputated yet he is a very joyful person. He's always got a story to tell me. You

---

7. Luke 15:11-32

might say, "Well, he's nuts, he's crazy," but he definitely is not and, in fact, he is a very reasonable guy. I asked him once, "How come you're always so patient and always in such a good mood?" He answered, "God is good. Very, very good." For him, that's a reality. I know it's not just words. I know because he's patient and kind.

That just knocks my socks off. Here I am, doing my job as a physician and I am getting paid for the privilege of listening to him. I should be paying him!

My faith plays a big role in the way I talk with patients but sometimes conflicts arise. A patient of mine who is HIV positive comes in thinking she might be pregnant. Her pregnancy test comes back positive. I ask how she feels about it.

In such situations I always hope very much that she'll say, "Well, it's good news but I'm scared. Can my baby be healthy?" Then I can explain that actually there is good news for her. Yes, she can have a healthy baby. If she takes her medications and has some support, the chances are overwhelming that she'll have a healthy baby without HIV. I can't predict the future, but with the phenomenal medicines we have to suppress this virus, I can tell her that she has a 99.99 percent chance of having a healthy baby. She needs to know that it really is reasonable to hope for this, and we can help her achieve it.

On the other hand, I'm scared of hearing from the woman, "This is really bad news. I want an abortion." In my experience, when a woman says that, her mind's made up. If she wants an abortion I have to tell her, "Gosh, I can't help you with that. If you decided to have your baby, we can give you lots of help. We can help with housing or other forms of support. Please give us a call if you decide to continue the pregnancy. Otherwise you need to go talk to someone else about that choice." When a woman responds with total rejection, it's depressing and tragic.

We see plenty of substance abusers reject help. Folks who are "using" are usually in bad relationships. They're making bad choices, which are inherently self-destructive. When this is the case with a patient, you try to help them from the margin by showing your concern and care. To directly attack the core of the problem may drive them away. You tell them, "There is treatment. You can go to a 12-step meeting today. There's help for you. There's counseling." As a physician you want to help them stop being self-destructive and often that approach speaks to them. They need to know that you want to see them back again.

It's very important to keep people engaged in their own care and that's a challenge. When someone's using drugs, we can see that it's bad for them. When someone's in sexual relationships with multiple partners, it's bad from a health point of view, as well as from a social and emotional point of view. We are called to keep people engaged and to continually suggest to them what they can do to change and where they can get support and help.

Take the situation of a patient with emphysema who still smokes. They're on oxygen and yet they're still smoking. Do you say, "I'm not going to care for you"? No, that's not going to help the patient. Do you say, "Well, I'm burned out. I'm not going to mention quitting smoking again"? Well, that's not going to help the patient either.

So sometimes you rail at the patient; sometimes you joke with them. Maybe you raise your voice a little. But you must always show them care and concern. To help the patient quit smoking you might try the patches, the lozenges, medications—you try this and that. You might not make a point of mentioning their habit every time you see them but maybe at least every other time. In the end you may try more than 10 different strategies to help get them to stop. Above all, you try to convince them to keep trying.

God doesn't ask us to change other people's behavior. He only asks us to change our own. As physicians, our job isn't to change people, but God does ask us to keep suggesting to people, in caring, loving ways, that they are invited to change their behavior. It's tough and challenging. In fact, it keeps the practice of medicine exciting.

I'm a big fan of the insightful writer M. Scott Peck, a Christian psychiatrist and author of *The Road Less Traveled* and *People of the Lie*. He asks why it is that when we continually offer people an opportunity to change, some do it and others don't. At first, he thought that maybe if it's hard or painful to change, people will say no, and if it's easy, they'll say yes. But that's not the case. Some people endure a lot of pain and it's hard, but they want to do it, they're willing to take on that struggle and to endure. Others don't even want to think about making changes. It's hard to know why that is. One factor is grace.

Scott Peck is saying that we don't know who might change, or how and why. It's not our job to figure that out. Our job is to continually offer the opportunity for change and then wait and see what happens. We need to keep reminding others that even if they don't seem to be loved by anyone, God loves them and they can be forgiven. What an amazing thing, to be forgiven.

It's worth repeating that changing people is not our job. If you think it's your job to change the patient and the patient does change, you may mistakenly take the credit when it's not yours. And if the patient doesn't change, you may get frustrated. And if you get frustrated, you're good for about a year before you burn out. Nobody can endure that kind of frustration for long. The way to endure professionally is to realize that we're not supposed to be changing people; we're supposed to be caring for people. In different ways, we are there to make it clear to patients that there is help and that they are loved. This kind of attitude helps a lot in dealing with patients' foibles and failures.

In my professional career, I've worked with HIV patients and substance abusers. I've also worked in prisons, directed clinical research, and taught. I've received a few awards, such as the Community Health Leadership Award from the Robert Wood Johnson Foundation. That came with $100,000; it was one heck of an award! I used the money to found the Star Kids Scholarship Program, which provides tuition, uniforms and tutoring for children whose parents have been incarcerated or suffered from substance abuse. The Star Kids Program operates in Newport County, Rhode Island and Fall River and New Bedford, Massachusetts.

These kids are hurting "big time" and are at risk of dropping out of school. There's an intergenerational cycle of incarceration for those children when they get older. But we've got something that can help these kids a lot: mission-based schools. Some of the schools are Catholic; others are charter schools, private or Christian. Tuition at these schools is often cheap, so our scholarships go a long way. Many children whose parents are in jail or come from the inner city and difficult families thrive in mission-based schools. The schools provide a great sense of community and continuity, especially when a child can attend the same school from kindergarten through eighth grade.

I have been fortunate to have success in my life, but that success comes at a price. Success breeds arrogance, impatience, and being short-tempered. And I am frequently accused of all three of those things! It's too easy when you're multitasking to just tell rather than to ask somebody to do something. But life has its ways of showing you that this is not very nice.

We all have to struggle sometimes to find balance in our lives—and balance is closely tied in with our calling, with what God is inviting us to do. To be honest, I don't have enough balance in my life. This morning, Luba, my hero and my best critic, told me, "You don't know how to say no." But I'm trying to find more balance. We go to Mass together on Sundays, which is great for us. We take trips with the kids—vacation trips, which are wonderful, but other trips too. I've gone twice to Haiti with my teenage son and daughter to work with the Missionaries of Charity, which is Mother Teresa's order. Haiti is a place of terrible hardship, now immensely worse following the recent earthquake. But to see the faces of the religious sisters in action is an awesome sight.

Luba and I have five children, who range in age from 7 to 21. They are our greatest blessing. The four oldest are our biological children, and we adopted our youngest, Nicholas, because Luba had had difficult pregnancies and was facing other risks because of age. Nicholas was 15 months old when he came to us from Ukraine. He has just turned seven and has been a bundle of joy. The adoption process is a lot like pregnancy; you're not sure exactly what God's going to give you. It's a beautiful grace, a gift, just slightly different from having a biological child. Our kids are fortunate to go to Catholic school, which is a big help. The school helps them to see the spiritual side of reality and to remain Catholic in a secular world.

One afternoon a week, I teach a course on C. S. Lewis at Brown University, which is proof that I have trouble saying no. I've been a fan of Lewis since college. Teaching the class was my response to the 50-year itch. When you turn 50, it's so easy to get into trouble, especially if you're a guy. So when I turned 50, I read Lewis's Space Trilogy for the first time.[8] I thought it was wonderful stuff, about the great adventure of life and how we're all invited by God to participate. Early in his career, Lewis wrote mostly didactic works and commentary, but later he came to the conclusion that a writer can be much more convincing to readers by presenting an entertaining invention through fiction.

In the course, we read both his fiction and non-fiction (including *The Screwtape Letters*, *The Problem of Pain*, and *A Grief Observed*) and we watch the film version of *Shadowlands*. We have great discussions, led by the students, who are at all different places spiritually. Not everybody agrees, but we talk about what Lewis is

---

8. *Out of the Silent Planet* (first published in 1938), *Perelandra* (1943), and *That Hideous Strength* (1945).

trying to say. Halfway through the class, we stop for tea because it's the middle of the afternoon, and, since we are studying an Englishman, it would be wrong not to.

Right now I'm also in the first year of a discernment program for the diaconate. I have been thinking and praying about this for a while, and although I still don't have a clear answer, my hope is that my calling and vocation will unfold and develop over time. The whole formation process for deacons takes four years and requires a big time commitment. Some of the others in the program are ready to make that commitment but I'm not there yet. I missed last Monday's meeting and I'm going to miss this Monday's. I have to figure out if I'm really being called to reorganize my life in a way to make it work.

In some ways I'm scared to death of being a deacon. Most deacons work in a parish church assisting the priest. I go with my family to Mass every Sunday, but right now my involvement in parish life is not very deep. The idea of working in parish ministry is uncomfortable for me. Prison ministry or ministry with those in substance abuse treatment is appealing but when a deacon is ordained, he swears obedience to his bishop just as a priest does. So if the bishop says you've got to go here or there, you've got to go; if you don't like it, "Tough luck." I just have to leave a lot of this up to God.

We're not good at evangelization in the Catholic Church. We don't know how to do it nor are we comfortable with it. But it's clear if you read The Book, you've got to evangelize. It's not optional; it's mandatory.

I would love it if the Church were able to reach out more effectively to folks who are marginalized. People are often struggling and they are asking for and are open to help. My sense is that the Catholic Church has much to offer. For example, when you've been using drugs you feel terrible inside. For the addict, the grace of forgiveness is really powerful. Telling someone who's a heroin or cocaine user that Jesus died for them and their sins are forgiven is a big, big deal. If we're not telling these people about salvation, that's a problem. What could be more important?

But those who need to hear about Jesus often aren't told. Or maybe it is being said, but not often enough. Part of the problem is that the Catholic Church is stretched too thin. When there are more priests and nuns, the Church is better able to work in marginalized communities. But today, there are fewer priests and fewer religious.[9] If a single priest is taking care of two parishes, he doesn't have time to celebrate Mass at a local substance abuse program. There are only so many hours in a day. It's a challenge.

There are only so many hours in the day for me as well. If I become a deacon, can I work as a physician full-time? I don't think so. I probably need to work half-time in medicine and half-time in the diaconate. There are a lot of good infectious disease doctors around but not many people who are comfortable working in prisons or around cocaine users. I've been doing this for 20 years and I'm comfortable with it. Do I have the calling?

God asks all of us to be workers in the Vineyard and obviously there are thousands of ways we can do that. But I ask: Who is in the Vineyard working with people who have substance abuse issues? Or with those in prison who have not heard Christ's message of love and mercy? Who is telling these people about Mary, His Mother, and her great love for us, her offer to help us at two in the morning when we are anxious and upset, her efforts to lead us to her Son? How about me?

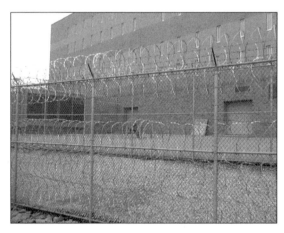

Rhode Island Department of Corrections

— Ad Majorem Dei Gloriam —

---

9. For those readers who may be non-Catholic, the word "religious" when it is used as a noun, as in this case, refers to monks and nuns.

3

Dr. Richard Shoup

CLOSING
THE CIRCLE

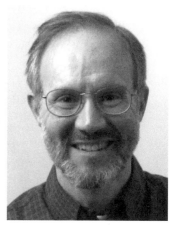

I'm eternally grateful to my parents for raising me to believe in God even though at times it was a struggle. I was born in Pennsylvania, and during my childhood, my parents and I worshipped in the Presbyterian Church. We moved around Pennsylvania several times during my childhood because of my father's work. When I was about 12 years old, we moved back to the family stomping grounds in Ellington, Connecticut, a small rural town where my father's mother had been born and raised. At that point we began attending the Congregational Church.

At the time we moved back there, Ellington was really changing. It had been very rural with many dairy farms. I remember doing a report on the town in high school. At the time, the town's population was 7,707—a number that stuck in my head. Today, the population is easily double that. Most of the farms have gone out of business because it's so hard to be a small farmer these days. All that once flat, gorgeous, fertile farmland is being turned into subdivisions.

I went to the public high school in Ellington, as did my wife. I was convinced that after I graduated high school I would never come back; I would leave town and that would be it. Well, I did go away to college, but apart from that, I haven't left Ellington since.

In my senior year in high school, I started asking a lot of the big questions: Who am I? What is the fullness of truth? What is the true nature of the universe? I ended up, figuratively speaking, walking down church row and asking questions. Among them was this: How do you pick out a church from among all these choices? I didn't know it then, but there are at least 25,000 denominations of Protestantism.

As I was going through this process, I made a connection with a teacher in high school who was serious about things religious. He was also, by far, one of the best teachers we had in the school. He had a Ph.D. and could teach almost any subject as well as, or even better than, the other teachers. His name was Evan Lawn. In freshman year, Dr. Lawn taught my Government class. As a sophomore and junior he taught me Geometry and Alegbra II. Senior year he oversaw a program for the academically gifted of which I was a part, which included AP European History and English.

One day at school I asked Dr. Lawn, "Why do you believe in God?" He told me, "You know I can't answer that question in a public school. But you're welcome to come to my house and talk." That was the start of my big adventure. At first we talked mostly about why, specifically, he believed in God. His answer was that it's a lot easier to believe in God if you can see some sort of objective signs of His existence. At that point, I didn't think such a thing was possible. But through a series of conversations with Dr. Lawn, my mind began to change.

The pivotal truth for me was the incorrupt body of St. Bernadette Soubirous, the visionary who was visited by Our Lady at Lourdes. Dr. Lawn introduced me to the miracle of her body's preservation from decay. My reasonably good science background told me that this was an occurrence that couldn't happen in the natural order of things. A person dies; their body decays. When St. Bernadette's body had been dug up her flesh had not decayed and was even supple. Yet the rosary, with which she had been buried, had rusted away. That was very striking to me.

I also learned about apparitions of the Virgin Mary to Bernadette when she was a young girl, and about the many miracles associated with Lourdes. Dr. Lawn told me about the spring that appeared when Bernadette began digging in the ground, and about how many people have been healed after going to Lourdes and drinking or touching the water from that very spring. Many things that couldn't happen in nature began to flood together in my mind. These things told me very strongly that God existed in ways I previously could not have conceived.

Anyway, that got me started. I began to visit Catholic churches from time to time, just to be with God. Throughout the summer I continued to visit and talk with Dr. Lawn. In the fall I went off to Dartmouth College and there I continued to explore. I read books Dr. Lawn recommended and talked to the campus Catholic chaplain, Monsignor Nolan. A remarkable priest, he had gotten a Catholic student center started just off campus, which gave me a place to go and talk with people. Chief among them was Sheila Flanigan, the sister of my friend and classmate, Tim.[10] She and I talked a lot and shared stories, and she recommended more books I could read. A lot of us would go to the center to study in the evenings. Every evening at five o'clock they had a Mass for students. Some faculty members would attend as well. At 10 o'clock there was a study break, and we'd all say the rosary.

The Catholic student center provided a context in which I could begin looking at things Catholic. I think some of the other students were surprised at me. I was not yet a member of the Catholic Church but I was certainly hanging around a lot and acting pretty interested. I guess you could have called me something of a "Catholic wannabe." The thing that held me back from conversion was my parents' vehement objection. It was very hard on them; they felt betrayed and even disgusted.

I really think my mother had the hardest time putting it together. She had lived for many years in a mining town in Pennsylvania, where the Catholics were coal miners and hard drinkers. To put it mildly, they apparently didn't set the highest moral example. So I think that colored my mother's perception of Catholic life. She thought that I was giving up everything she had raised me to believe. But nothing could have been further from the truth. Ironically, every time I came to understand a different aspect of Catholic teaching, it was as if a light would come on. I felt like I was completing, rather than rejecting, what I had been raised to believe.

For example, as a Protestant I had been taught that the Bible was it, the ultimate authority for Christian teaching. But in digging into the history and origins of the Bible, I realized that it didn't just drop from heaven. It was the Church councils that approved the canon of the Bible.[11] The process involved a group of men making decisions guided by the Holy Spirit. And those men were Catholic; at that time in history, all Christians were Catholic.

In addition, I began to see that both Scripture and Tradition are essential for the Christian life. Tradition comes out of Scripture

---

10. Dr. Timothy Flanigan is the subject of Chapter 2 of this book.
11. In the year 393, the African Synod of Hippo approved the canon of the New Testament and the Septuagint books of the Old Testament. This decision was further ratified by the Councils of Carthage in 397 and 419.

and Scripture is informed by Tradition. One is not greater than the other, but they are intimately intertwined and hold each other together. As I came to understand this, Scripture actually took on greater importance for me. This knowledge enriched my insight into passages of Scripture and ways of looking at the Bible that I had grown up with.

The view of the Catholic Church towards the Bible really impressed me. The Church took the words of the Bible much more seriously than anything I had seen growing up. There comes a point where, if you really believe the Scripture is the word of God and is inspired by the Holy Spirit, then you pay serious attention to every word. You pay attention to the translation, to where those words come from, because the nuances of the words in a translation can dramatically affect the meaning.

For example, the so-called *Good News Bible* is really a businessman's paraphrase. People think it's a translation, but it's not. If you compare those words to the Greek of the New Testament and the Hebrew of the Old Testament, there's a drastic difference between what the original text says and what the so-called translation says. The way something is translated takes on a huge, huge significance.

During my freshman year at Dartmouth I kept talking with my former teacher, Dr. Lawn, who had become a close friend. I spent time delving deeply into the Bible, taking it more seriously than ever before. I also spent time with God, in prayer and meditation. I even tried to be received into the Church at Dartmouth. But Monsignor Nolan wasn't too keen on that idea. My parents were still very much against my conversion and he didn't want to cause trouble with them.

In the summer of 1976, when I got back home to Ellington, I went to talk to Dr. Lawn. He told me about several students from my old high school who had decided to join him the next year in private study of the Scriptures. The more he told me about it, the more I wanted to do it too. So four of us put aside our other commitments and studied for a year with Dr. Lawn. We studied the Bible in its original languages, in Greek and Hebrew, and in translation. We spent time reading the writings of the Church Fathers and learning about the lives of the saints.

That turned out to be a wonderful year for me. I lived with Dr. Lawn and his wife in their home, where the four of us students led a life of study and prayer, daily Mass and daily rosary, adoration of the Blessed Sacrament and other devotions. We were assisted by Dr. Lawn's father-in-law, Moses Bailey, who had retired from his position as a professor of the Old Testament at the Hartford Theological Seminary. An unusually bright man and a wonderful scholar, he taught us Hebrew and Latin. He certainly thought Catholics were wrong-minded, but he was willing enough to work with us, and he seemed interested to have eager students.

My parents had pretty much given up on me. It was awful for them that I was taking a year off from school to do this, of all things. They were disgusted with what I was doing and it was very hard on all of us. But I was following the life I had to follow. On December 8 of that year, on the feast of the Immaculate Conception, I was received into the Church.

No one from my family came to the ceremony. But I was received at the same time as my parents' next-door neighbor, Fran, who was of my parents' generation. When I was in high school, I had been her paperboy. Fran was pretty gregarious, and I would go over to her house and talk about God with her and her husband. She ended up coming into the Catholic Church through Dr. Lawn's influence, just as I did.

It was so hard to go against my parents' wishes and to see the rift that it caused. But I had developed such a strong conviction that the Church held the fullness of truth that I had to act on it. Not to do so would have been to betray my most fundamental beliefs. You have to act on what you see and know, because if you don't, you're lost. I had to do this, no matter what. My parents could very well have disowned me and put me out of their lives. They didn't go that far, but I was prepared for that, because I had to follow what God had shown me to the exclusion of everything else. It wasn't always easy, but in one sense, when the truth is that clear, you *have* to follow it.

I had planned to go back to Dartmouth the next year. But my parents were so upset at what I had done that, when I approached them about college, they said, "We're not going to help you." So I had no funds for college. I ended up staying a second year and studying with Dr. Lawn. This was an unexpected turn of events, but it proved to be very fruitful. By the end of my second year at Dr. Lawn's, I was considered by the college to be independent of my parents. That opened up all kinds of financial aid and I received a scholarship that enabled me to go back and complete my under-graduate degree.

I had started college as a pre-med student, but when I returned I chose a double major in classics (Greek and Latin) and classical archeology. This was a great combination of studies and I loved it. I really wanted to study the sweep of history through Western civilization, so I started with the Greeks and Romans. At that time I had thought that I might be headed for the seminary, and so studying Greek and Latin made sense to me.

I also took courses in medieval history and was actually only a few courses short of a third major in history. And I think if I'd had the time I would have stayed in school and majored in a few other things, such as art history. It wasn't the standard path to medical school, but I don't regret any of my college studies. The archeology part was particularly fascinating for me. I spent a semester in Rome, which was marvelous on all counts. I saw a lot of Roman ruins and Greek ruins as well, since some of the best-preserved Greek ruins in the world are in Italy. And I also got to visit many wonderful Catholic shrines in the process.

By that time I was very much in the Catholic Church. When I walked into St. Peter's Basilica for the first time, a very strong sensation came over me that this was my true home. It was a surprisingly intimate experience to have in this, the biggest church in the world. I spent a fair amount of time at St. Peter's and got to know one of the priests who lived in the Vatican. He took me on a personal tour that included a visit to the tomb of St. Peter.

I was in Rome shortly after John Paul II became Pope. I didn't understand the significance of his election at the time. The fact that the College of Cardinals had just elected a Polish cardinal as Pope, after centuries of Italians, was quite a shock to the world, but the drama of that shift didn't register with me. I just thought, "Okay, he's Polish."

I think my eventual understanding of the papacy itself was an outright gift from God. It wasn't something I approached academically, looking through the Scriptures for explanations and justifications. It was almost as if I woke up one morning and said to myself, "This makes sense." I didn't have to struggle with it. I think maybe God said, "Let's give it to him. He's not going to get this on his own."

When I left high school, my original career plans had leaned toward becoming a physician. After I became a Catholic though, I began to wonder if I wasn't being called to the priesthood or religious life. As I finished my last three years of college and spent more time trying to discern my calling, it became clearer to me that the religious or consecrated life wasn't my vocation. In retrospect, I kind of wonder if I would have even remained Catholic if I had tried to enter the seminary since back in the 1970s, some of the seminaries were in pretty bad shape.

In the days when I was thinking of med school, I also wondered about becoming a medical missionary. I had grown up hearing about Dr. Albert Schweitzer's medical mission work and I had a very high regard for him. He was a natural role model for me, because like him, I was also an organist. I had learned to play piano as a child and I worked as a church organist right out of college. In fact, I used some of Schweitzer's editions of Bach organ music when I played at church. But in the end, I just didn't think I was called to the life of a missionary.

After I finished college, I went back to Ellington and finally realized I wanted to be a physician, more than I wanted to teach or to do anything else. My undergraduate coursework was insufficient for med school, so I commuted to Wesleyan University in Middletown and took additional science courses.

I believed then, and still believe now, that a liberal education is important. The liberal arts are designed to liberate the mind and I had wanted to soak up as much of that as I could in college. But I also loved studying the sciences at Wesleyan. I think it's interesting that most people believe you gain more spiritual enrichment from the humanities than from the sciences. But in my experience, that's not necessarily the case. Take calculus, for example. I don't have a mathematical mind, but after studying calculus for a year, I discovered it is really remarkable stuff. That course gave me a strong sense of beauty, both the beauty of math as a natural science and the beauty of creation. I now see mathematics as a gorgeous aspect of creation.

Physics speaks to the beauty of creation as well. I remember at one point looking at the theory of relativity: $E=mc^2$. As we worked on that equation in class, the fact that energy and matter are interchangeable, it suddenly struck me: Holy smokes—our existence depends entirely on a continual act of the will of God! Years later, I discovered that this was a part of Catholic teaching. Einstein's theory of relativity opened that up and made it clear to me. So there are lots of treasures in the natural sciences.

After I finished my required courses, I spent the better part of a year while I was applying to med school working as a lab technician at Rockefeller University in New York City. It was a small medical research institute, packed with Nobel laureates, who were an amazing, intense group of scientists. When I applied for the job, I didn't know that. I was just looking at it as a place to work.

My girlfriend, Marie, was also living in New York City at the time, only on the other side of town. We had gone to high school together in Ellington and she was in Columbia University's nursing school. So we got to see each other, but not a lot. It's funny; you would think if you lived in the same city, you'd get to visit each other a lot. But it would take more than an hour for me to travel from my side of Manhattan to hers.

By December of that year I had been accepted into the medical school at the University of Connecticut. I was also thinking about proposing to Marie. A lot of my thinking seemed to crystallize at this point, so I withdrew all of my other medical school applications and chose UConn. That June, Marie and I got married and in August I started med school.

When I was a medical student, I really loved surgery. I like working with my hands—it's something that comes easily and naturally to me. So, to my wife's increasing trepidation, I looked closely at that specialty. Surgery requires rigorous training and is a very hard life. As I explored a few surgical residencies, I remember learning about one program that virtually boasted about having a 100 percent divorce rate among its surgical residents. I thought, "If that's how the program treats its residents and that's what's expected of me, I certainly don't want that residency. My family is way too important to me."

One of the surgical residents I met during my training told me, "You know, Rich, if you can do anything else but surgery, do it. If you can't, then you've got to be a surgeon." That was a clear way of putting it. And that's how I ended up choosing internal medicine. From there, I got really interested in pulmonary medicine because that specialty combined office work and critical care work. I liked the human physiology of the specialty and the opportunity to work with my hands doing various procedures—not really to the extent that a surgeon does, but enough to satisfy me and still provide a reasonable family life.

That next year was fast-paced. Marie had graduated from nursing school and was working as a pediatric nurse at Hartford Hospital, while I was grinding away at med school. We had our first child—an experience that, as any parent knows, is unbelievably profound. It's really kind of interesting that during my second year in med school, I didn't study such long hours, because now I had a son as well as a wife. But somehow I think I was more focused, and I did better than I had done in my first year. Actually, it seemed as if with each child we had, I was more effective in my studies.

We really worked on keeping our faith alive in our family life. With the arrival of our first child, I felt a tremendous responsibility before God: Here was another soul entirely dependent on my care. I began to understand from the start that part of my role as a parent was to help this child get into heaven. Perhaps that was what focused my thinking so sharply. So as a family, we started having regular devotions together. I also used to gather with some friends to pray the Liturgy of the Hours at the UConn Medical School chapel in Farmington.

Medical school was very intense and so was my three-year medical residency. Then I decided to sub-specialize in pulmonary critical care—that was another three years. At each step, I would look around at other training programs in the region to see what my options were. Each time I decided to stay at UConn. That was partially because of the strong family ties; my family and Marie's both lived in the area. Marie was from a family of six kids, five of whom stayed in Ellington. The one who "moved away" is only 20 minutes away in Windham. Marie's family is quite close, and it was nice for our kids to be around so many cousins. We were grateful too, for the family support.

I was introduced to sleep medicine during my pulmonary training. One of the doctors I worked with, Dr. Richard Castriatta, started the sleep lab at Mount Sinai Hospital in Hartford and has gone on to head the sleep program at Baylor University in Texas. I got a thorough introduction to the field through him and when it came time to do a six-month elective during my pulmonary rotation, I spent the entire time learning sleep medicine.

Many of my career choices have been based on what's best for my family life. In fact, as I went looking for jobs in my field, I didn't bother looking farther than Connecticut. I'd done that several times before and had just ended up staying in Ellington. After my training was complete, I contacted several local pulmonary groups and told them that I was from the area, wanted to stay here and was in the market for a position. None of them was advertising, but somehow doors opened and people were willing to talk with me, partly, perhaps, because they knew I *wanted* to be here. I finally accepted a position at an office in Vernon, Connecticut, adjacent to my hometown of Ellington. I did inpatient work at nearby Manchester Hospital and they put me in charge of the sleep unit, which they were just getting started. Over time, the sleep medicine part of my practice got busier and busier and after a couple of years, I found myself doing entirely sleep medicine.

I work by day, but the technologists on my staff work by night. Patients with suspected sleep disorders come to our lab for a "sleep study" or polysomnogram in which they spend the night sleeping under closely monitored conditions. Then either my associate or I interpret the sleep study data. We also spend a lot of time with each patient and get to know them fairly well. A sleep study is necessary for a proper diagnosis. A patient might present with a series of symptoms that seems to indicate sleep apnea, but the study might indicate little or no apnea. Yet the patient is sleepy. So you start sorting out what else might be going on. A fairly long list of things can cause sleepiness, with sleep apnea being the most common, but not the only possibility. You have to verify the diagnosis rather than work on assumptions.

When you look at a sleep study of a patient who is severely affected by sleep apnea, it's really striking to watch the breathing pauses that occur, sometimes over 100 times an hour. You can see the oxygen levels plummet and see the heart race, and with each new series of breaths, the heart picks up again and then slows. When you look at what happens and understand the physiology, you realize how nasty sleep apnea is. And when you talk to some of these patients, you find that they're dragging through the day. I've seen people fall asleep in mid-conversation. I've had wives tell me stories like the one about a guy who was standing up and talking, then leaned back against a wall, and suddenly fell asleep. Sleep apnea increases the risk of motor vehicle accidents, hypertension, heart disease, and sudden death.

In sleep medicine you get to use all your medical training. The field involves a combination of intellectual and academic disciplines, along with a very human aspect. That's what is most interesting to me. People come in all stripes and they all present unique challenges. I spend a lot of time helping people understand what is actually happening in their sleep. I often say that people with sleep apnea are the last to know about it, since they're "sleeping" through it. But even though they are desperately trying to, they still cannot sleep well. Their spouses may have known for years that something was wrong, yet it can be hard for these patients to accept. But in most cases, once they're effectively treated, they come back and say, "Wow, what a difference!"

Treatment for sleep apnea might involve a CPAP machine,[12] which blows air through the upper airway to prevent it from closing off. Or it may involve a dental device that acts like a retainer after braces, to pull the lower jaw forward. Obesity is often a cause. The surge in sleep apnea in this country has closely followed the surge in obesity. So we end up working with a lot of our patients to encourage the weight loss that is the one thing that can cure this ailment. The machine can control the apnea, but if you can cure it, that's even better.

It's really wonderful to be able to help someone with sleep apnea, to successfully treat them so they can live a normal life again. In some cases, it can help people keep their livelihood. For example, a truck driver who has sleep apnea might not be safe on the road until he's treated. My goal in such cases is to get the patient back to work as quickly as possible, but also to make sure he's safe. And typically, once he's treated, he's fine. It can be very rewarding to make that kind of difference in a person's life.

I try to pattern my practice on the Franciscan model. With both the patients I treat and the staff members with whom I work, I try to remember that everyone is made in the image and likeness of God, and as such, deserves respect. Unless you take the time to think about that, it's easy to forget, and you can get careless. So I try to treat each person before me as if they were Christ. It's hard to get upset with somebody when you think of that person as the image of Christ. I try my best to figure out how I can help that person. Do I remember this with every patient? Hardly. Do I want to remember with every patient? Yes I do.

St. Francis of Assisi is said to have taught: "Preach the Gospel at all times and when necessary use words." That quote is so apt, because what you do conveys more than what you say. My ideal is to remember that quote every time I walk in to meet with a patient or talk to my staff. It's the way I think all people should be treated.

Back when I was doing pulmonary medicine and critical care, I had a series of patients who made me realize how dependent we all are on God. I was treating patients who were critically ill on ventilators in the intensive care unit. I tried to help their families

---

12. Continuous Positive Airway Pressure machine

through the crisis of not knowing whether their loved one would survive or die. Seeing that, and being so intimately a part of that, it was just natural for me to turn to God. I do everything I can as a doctor—there's no question about that. But even the best doctor in the world can't keep someone alive when it's their time to go. When they are right at the interface between life and death, so many patients could easily go either way. What happens at that point is whatever God has ordained.

With sleep medicine, obviously, the challenges are not nearly as intense as pulmonary critical care. But I still get some tough cases. I had one patient, David, who was perfectly capable of sleeping, but increasingly chose not to sleep. His sleep pattern became erratic. He would stay up late working at hobbies until sleep overpowered him for a short period. His wife used to find him asleep at odd times and places in the house, such as the family room floor. Because of his disordered sleep habits, David became increasingly unable to function.

The first time I spoke to David and his wife, I had to figure out a way to convince him to devote some time each day to sleep. It is strange to say but I had to convince him that sleep was as essential to life as eating and drinking. I tried suggesting that he set aside a certain length of time each day for sleep. I think I initially proposed six hours, but he and his wife both said, "Oh, that's entirely too much!" They were intelligent people but had come to accept as normal the fact that David didn't sleep. I finally got him to commit to two hours of sleep each night. Some time later, when David came back to see me, he had gotten back on track. He had been falling asleep for increasingly longer stretches of time. He was now able to function around the house, interact with his family, and able to drive again without scaring his wife to death. It would have been easy to give up on someone like that. But I feel an obligation with every patient to say a silent prayer asking God's help to try to figure out how best to care for that person.

To live as a serious Christian, it doesn't matter what you do for a living. What does matter is that you shape your work with your Christianity. In my case, that means shaping my sleep medicine practice with my Christian faith, treating others as if they were Christ.

At home I have tried to be faithful to Christ as well. My wife, Marie, and I sought out a parish that was pretty serious about its Catholicism and worshipped in a way that reflected that attitude.

We had devotions with the children every night when they were young. As the kids were growing up, we read aloud a wonderful series of books on the saints, which they loved. And since we read them together, I think it helped all of us remember how important our faith is—that it's not just an added attraction, but a gift and part of everything we do.

At one stage, about the time our oldest child was in seventh grade, we were struggling because the kids were losing their excitement about the Faith. I was concerned, but I didn't quite know what to do about it. We needed something more. We attended an East Coast Catholic Conference and heard three interesting speakers, Jerry and Gwen Coniker, along with Cardinal Francis Arinze, who was a member of the Curia of the Vatican. The Conikers had started a group called the Apostolate for Family Consecration with Cardinal Arinze as a close advisor. They spoke to the conference about their work. At the time, I had made a mental note of it, but that was about it.

Soon we received a mailing from the Apostolate about a place called Catholic Familyland. The brochure invited families to spend a week there together in the summer as vacation-time but also as a way to renew their faith by attending Mass daily and studying the Catechism. The concept reminded me very much of the Protestant church camps that I had enjoyed when I was growing up. I managed to talk Marie into going and we packed up our tent and camping gear and drove with the kids to Bloomingdale, Ohio, where Familyland was located. We'd set out with a little trepidation; we were traveling 10 hours away based just on a brochure.

We ended up falling in love with Familyland. We found ourselves in the midst of dozens of families from all over the county, all of whom were very serious about their Catholicism. And our kids were suddenly with a large group of children their own age whose parents were as "crazy" as we were, so they didn't feel out of place. All at once, they began to realize that there was a whole lot to this Faith. Familyland, which attracted between 500 and 750 people for four week-long sessions, had wonderful age-appropriate programs for kids and phenomenal evening sessions for teens that helped them learn more about their faith and have fun in the process.

Our oldest son, John Paul, was especially impressed by the kids he'd met. He told us, "Those kids really know their Catechism. They're homeschooled. I would like to do that too." Marie and I had toyed with the idea but hadn't really considered it seriously until our son made that pronouncement. And as soon as his sister Mary found out what he'd said, she told us, "Well, you can't do him and not me!" So suddenly my wife was in the business of homeschooling. John Paul homeschooled for one year. Mary homeschooled from sixth to eighth grade. Ben started in the sixth grade and Clare in the third. All headed to Catholic high school after eighth grade.

While homeschooling, we made use of a lot of the catechetical materials from the Apostolate for Family Consecration. Their materials are very interactive and cover all the basics. They were developed for large families, in which the children range in age from 3 to 17. You can teach a concept to the youngest child with pictures, then turn to papal documents that teach the same concept at the level of the oldest child. Each lesson poses a series of questions that allow you to delve deeper into the subject, using documents from Vatican II and encyclicals. Several well-known teachers have taped educational videos for the Apostolate's library, including Cardinal Arinze and Mother Teresa of Calcutta, who were both on the Apostolate's board of advisors.

Our visit to Familyland was the start of really strengthening ties within our family and enriching what we had together in terms of our faith. Our kids keep in touch with the friends they made at Familyland—instant messaging them. We liked Familyland so much that we now go there for a week each summer and to their fall conference as well. They are able to get some great speakers for the conference because Familyland is only half an hour from Franciscan University of Steubenville. We had been looking for support in our efforts to be serious about what our Faith teaches and Familyland has been tremendously nourishing.

To nurture my own faith I go to Mass every day, which is a huge treasure in and of itself. Many days, the two children who are still here at home with us accompany me to Mass before I drive them to school. Often we pray together as a family, though it has gotten harder because the kids' schedules are all over the place. Sometimes the best I can do is say the rosary as I'm driving to the office. On the way home, I'll pray the Divine Mercy Chaplet. I try to fit in some kind of devotional reading during the day. And, of course, our family always goes to Mass on Sundays. I believe you have to feed the Faith.

When the kids were growing up, we'd read out loud to them, and we do that even now from time to time. J.R.R. Tolkien has long been one of our favorite authors. More recently, we've read *The Shadow of His Wings*, by Gereon Goldmann. It's the striking story of a German priest who, as a seminarian, was conscripted into the German army during the Nazi regime. He tells an amazing tale of his experiences and how he was able to keep the Faith.

My parents and I are friends today. They still live here in Ellington and I go over to their house to visit. They are still not happy about my being Catholic but have just kind of accepted me. I think they're relieved that I got married instead of becoming a priest and they like my wife and their grandchildren.

About a year ago, my older daughter, Mary, entered a Capuchin convent in Pennsylvania that lives a very strict Franciscan life of utter poverty, chastity and obedience. They really live on the providence of God, and they're the happiest group of women I've ever met. They are dedicated to Christ with amazing joy and freedom. However, my daughter was only there for a couple of months when she got sick and had to leave. It was clear that God didn't want her in that community at that time and it's unclear whether she will eventually end up back there or whether God has something else in mind for her. My daughter's decision to enter the convent was yet another challenge for my parents. I tried explaining the concept, but that kind of life was totally foreign to them. It's one thing to be Catholic, but to follow a religious calling apart from the world is strikingly another thing.

Right now, Mary is studying biology at Eastern Connecticut State University, but she's planning to transfer out to Franciscan University in Steubenville, Ohio, to join her older brother, John Paul. Our younger son, Benedict, will follow them out there, assuming he gets in. The atmosphere at Franciscan is phenomenal. The school has a good academic program and fosters a strong spiritual life. My youngest biological daughter, Clare, is a student at the Academy of the Holy Family. And we also have a "foster daughter," Katrina, who is living with us while she studies at the University of Connecticut.

My oldest son, John Paul, wants to go into medicine. During spring break of his freshman year at Franciscan, he went on a medical mission to Ecuador sponsored by the University. The following year, he organized and ran another mission in Equador, and the year after that, he was put in charge of the entire mission program. So John Paul's pretty busy. He's not sure yet what specialty he plans to pursue, but tropical medicine sure looks interesting to him.

In April 2005, when Pope Benedict was elected, several friends called us saying, "Holy smokes, you have both Popes in your family!" John Paul II was Pope before my son John Paul was born, but Benedict XVI became Pope long after my son Benedict came along. I explained that we were very gratified as a family that the Holy See saw fit to follow our lead in choosing names.

We've come to feel a very special connection with Pope Benedict, which goes far beyond the name thing. Back when I was working at Rockefeller University, I met a woman named Christina from Italy who was doing post-doctoral work. She was a physician and a member of a group called Comunione e Liberazione (Communion and Liberation), a wonderful Catholic lay organization, founded by Monsignor Luigi Guissani. After working in New York, Christina returned to Italy and took vows and began living a consecrated life as part of the CL community in Rome while working as a doctor.

Some years later, we were able to go to Italy as a family, on a sort of vacation/pilgrimage, and we decided to see if we could get together with Christina. When we got to Rome, I called her and we arranged to meet outside the Vatican. "This is where I work now," she explained. She pointed up to the papal apartments and said, "That's where the Pope stays, and that next window is where I stay."

One of the women in Christina's community had been working for Cardinal Ratzinger before he was elected Pope. When this woman went to say goodbye to the new Pope as he was cleaning out his cardinal's desk, he asked her if she would help him organize the papal household. Traditionally nuns run the papal household, but as they talked about Comunione e Liberazione, it was decided that a group of these consecrated women would take on the job. Christina was invited to be part of this group, to which she quickly said yes.

To hear Christina talk about all this was really quite something. She had only started working in the papal household three weeks before our visit. She told us she was struck by how humble the Pope is and said she sees that humility in all aspects of his life. Christina gets to attend the Mass he offers every day, and they share a meal together. It's a very special relationship. Here she is, a doctor who ended up in the papal household. So, you never know as a physician where you're going to end up!

I still keep in touch with my old teacher, Evan Lawn. In fact, he lives in our in-law apartment. I still don't know exactly how that happened. He was closing up his house and was deciding where he was going to live. In the course of talking with Dr. Lawn about his plans, we began to discuss the space above the garage, and then one thing led to another. And somehow, we ended up adding an apartment to the house and Dr. Lawn moved in.

Dr. Lawn's 92 years old now, but he stays remarkably active and lives a very rich spiritual life. He comes and goes as he wishes, but I go to visit him regularly, to read Scripture with him and talk about spiritual things. He works and studies very intently and he has a lot of visitors, including a priest friend. To look at him, you'd guess he's in his 80s. To talk to the guy, you'd see that he is as sharp as ever. Just a few years back he taught himself Hebrew, and he loves to read the Bible in its original languages. I can follow some of it with him, and believe me, there's nothing like reading the original text of Scripture. The Hebrew text of the Old Testament is especially rich. It's a treasure most Christians have never tasted.

The in-law apartment is a bit of construction we never expected. But I guess in a way I've come full circle.

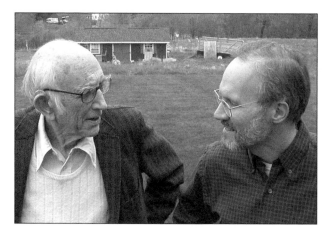

Dr. Evan Lawn and Dr. Richard Shoup

— *Ad Majorem Dei Gloriam* —

4

Dr. Paul Carpentier

A PASSION BORN OF THE SEA

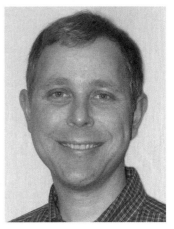

I grew up in a cozy little house on the village green in Charlton, Massachusetts. Charlton is a pretty rural town—we used to joke that there were more cows in town than people. The six of us kids in my family had the run of the neighborhood. All the neighborhood kids would gather for games of hide-and-seek, dodge ball, and hockey. We played football on the green, using shrubs to mark the goal lines. When we played baseball the town hall was our own Fenway Park Green Monster wall. One time we sent a high fly ball right through the third-story window of the town hall! We had to 'fess up, of course, but the batter was still credited with a home run.

I grew up in a Catholic family. I went to CCD and served as an altar boy, but the CCD class was a kind of mundane approach to Catholicism—with an emphasis on rules, regulations and the Ten Commandments. My dad owned a grocery store, but he was also very active in local politics, town projects, and community service. His store was the gathering place for people to stop in and discuss the town's problems. Dad was a real public servant. He served on building task forces for the police station and library and, as a planning board member, he was instrumental in assuring that women could be admitted to Bay Path, our regional vocational school. Dad worked especially hard for community-based services for mentally ill and disabled persons. Perhaps that was because my younger sister, Julie, was born with craniosynostosis and was disabled.[13]

But I had dreams of spending my life far from Charlton. As a child I loved watching *The Undersea World of Jacques Cousteau* on

---

13. Craniosynostosis is a congenital condition in which one or more of the sutures in an infant skull prematurely fuses resulting in restricted skull and brain growth.

television every month. Watching that show was a great thrill for me, seeing the exploration teams dive to study the wondrous depths of the sea. I wanted more than anything to be part of Jacques Cousteau's team.

My favorite class in fourth grade was mathematics, because I sat next to the bulletin board that held a poster depicting a cross-section of the ocean and its depths. Near the surface were a seagull, a whale surfacing to spout, and scuba divers swimming around. Deeper underneath the surface was a bathyscaphe surrounded by dolphins. Down in the darkness at the bottom of the sea were lantern fish and viperfish. I was enthralled. I thought to myself, "Every boy in the whole country probably wants to be on Jacques Cousteau's team—maybe even every boy in the whole world! If I want to get onto his team, I'd better do darn well in science and math. And I'd better study French too, because Jacques Cousteau speaks French." I went all the way through grade school and high school with that dream. It's good to have a dream even if it changes later, as mine did.

I went to Assumption College in Worcester, a landlocked school without a marine biology department. I held onto my dream, though. One of my professors told me years later that I seemed driven to excel in the sciences—driven by a dream. In the science department on campus I saw a poster for a program called SEA Semester, which involved six weeks of study on shore in Woods Hole on Cape Cod. After that, participants went out to sea for six weeks on the *Westward*, a 110-foot staysail schooner. I applied for the program and was thrilled when I was accepted. There on the schooner I actually caught and studied the lantern fish and viperfish whose pictures I had gazed at in fourth grade.

The program was rigorous, but when I had free time I went to my favorite place onboard—up on the yardarm—looking out over the ocean. And if I sat on the yardarm with my back against the foremast, I could see over the top of the foresail with the bowsprit stretching out in front of me, over the endless sea. I'd spend my spare moments up there, rocking back and forth with the waves, watching whales spout off in the distance, thinking, "This is beautiful, awesome! I love it here!" Yet a part of me felt ill at ease. My thoughts kept straying beyond the sea and marine biology. I couldn't help but wonder where my life was headed.

When I wasn't studying or pondering my future up on the yardarm, I'd be below decks writing letters to Suzanne, a wonderful young lady I had begun seeing at Assumption. In my letters I told her about my experiences on the trip but also about my dreams and uncertainty about the future. I had read the lives of the saints in college and had learned about Mother Teresa and her work with the poorest of the poor. At that time the famine in Somalia was in the news. I thought that maybe I could use a degree in marine biology to develop aquaculture that would grow food to feed the world's hungry people. But I also thought about the family doctor who had an office across the street from our home in Charlton. Dr. Achin, the only physician in town, provided such good and needed service for our community. I could hear God asking me, "Wouldn't you like to do something like that and be a family doctor?"

And something inside me answered, "Yes!"

As I was preparing to leave the *Westward*, I realized that I would not be going into marine biology after all. My trip on the schooner had been a wonderful gift but it was also the time God chose to tell me, "I've got other plans for your talents." I now see that the interest in marine biology was a gift to inspire me to excel in science.

So I applied to medical school but I found the whole selection process very disheartening. The interviews were brutal. They asked me, "Why do you want to go to med school?" I told them the truth—that I wanted to help people. My professors at Assumption had, of course, warned me not to say that—it's the stock answer, which they've heard a million times. One interview panel blatantly attacked my motives. Thinking they just wanted to test my resolve, I tried to answer them with energy and vigor. But they just came back at me harder. One doctor even yelled, "You're an insult to my office. Get out of here!" So I left, thinking, "I hope they were just testing me!"

When I went in for my interview at St. Louis University—my first choice—I was especially nervous. My research had told me that the program there was a patient-centered approach that viewed the patient as a whole person. Students did not learn to treat "the gallbladder in room 202," but rather "Mrs. Jones, who has three kids at home and who is presenting with a gallbladder attack." I knew that approach was the right fit for me.

"So," asked the dean of admissions, "your father runs a grocery store in a small town in Massachusetts?" "Yes," I answered eagerly "I've been working there since I was six years old, alongside my father and mother." I couldn't wait to tell him about what I wanted to do in medicine, about my dreams of caring for the whole patient. But he just shuffled through my paperwork and said, "Okay, thanks, see you later." I was heartbroken. Weeks went by and finally to my surprise SLU accepted me! On the day I got the letter of acceptance, I ran up to Suzanne, waving the letter and announcing, "I can help people!" And with that realization tears came to my eyes.

I felt fortunate to be accepted, but what about all those who had been rejected? I had many friends at Assumption, awesome people who would make dedicated, caring physicians, but wouldn't get a chance to serve because of their test scores. I was so mad on that first day of medical school, as I looked at the names on the lockers and thought of the applicants whose names were missing.

Before I began medical school, Suzanne and I were engaged. We thought a lot about our future together and started to ask some practical questions such as, "How many children will we have?" In the Bible it says, "Be fruitful and multiply; fill the earth and subdue it."[14] God loves children; He loves people. Doing the math, we could potentially have 16 children! Was that what God wanted? I brought that question to our med school chaplain, who uncharacteristically looked flustered and referred me to Father Dennis Brodeur, the head of the ethics program.

Father Dennis smiled and said, "Oh, you're talking about natural family planning." I didn't understand—though a cradle Catholic, I knew nothing about NFP. He explained, "A woman's cycle has windows of opportunity when she's fertile and when she is not, and a couple can rely on those windows to achieve or avoid pregnancy. By doing so, you're respecting your wife's body, your marriage and your future together, and she doesn't have to put chemicals in her body to suppress a good and natural system." "Wow," I said. "That sounds really powerful."

So when Suzanne and I got married and moved to St. Louis together, we took a class on NFP. Those classes turned my life and my career in a new direction and also proved to be incredibly valuable for our marriage. Not that we would necessarily have ended up divorced, but NFP helped keep us together through the stress of med school, through my residency when I was working 100 hours a week, and through all the other problems we had to face as a couple. We were able to concentrate on our relationship, knowing that we respected each other.

---

14. Genesis 1:28

Natural family planning is simple, effective, and easy to understand. It's inexpensive and it helps foster the marriage relationship, because it involves the husband and wife working together. The couple needs to take a class (not just read a book) to help them fully understand how to interpret the biomarkers of fertility that the woman's body gives her. The cervical mucus changes in consistency throughout the month. There's only a five-to-seven-day window in a typical month when a woman is fertile. By checking the mucus she can tell when that window is present. The couple keeps a daily record of the observations on a chart. Often the husband will do the charting, so that he is actively involved and both are aware of the approach of fertile periods.

With NFP, couples are empowered to achieve pregnancy or to sacrificially forgo intercourse to avoid pregnancy. The couple builds trust: If my spouse can abstain because it's a fertile time, then I know they can also faithfully abstain when we're apart, or when there's a medical reason to do so. They also enjoy a "honeymoon effect" after the times of abstaining. It means they have to keep talking. Is one spouse interested in intercourse even though it's a fertile time? Does that mean that spouse has decided a baby is more important than the reasons they had for waiting? NFP encourages communication. So many things don't get talked about when the birth control pill is used. But if a couple can talk about sex and cervical mucus, they can talk about anything.

When I first read Pope Paul VI's encyclical on human sexuality, marriage, and fertility, *Humanae Vitae* (*Of Human Life*), my response was "Now you're talking!" I saw it as so insightful, so obviously led by the Holy Spirit. The encyclical is not just a collection of rules and regulations, but a life-changing "yes" to what's good for us—our spouses, our children, our sexuality, and our relationships. The Pope recognized that contraception would radically change marital relationships and our approach to our sexuality and fertility. And what he envisioned has come to pass. Since the birth control pill was popularized, the divorce rate and the rate of abortions has increased rather than decreased. Single parent households, teen suicide, and child abuse are also all on the increase. If we can demean our fertility, the fruit of that fertility can be tossed aside. *Humanae Vitae* and the subsequent related encyclicals—*Evangelium Vitae*, *Donum Vitae*, and *Dignitas Personae*—are truly "love letters" from the Vatican sent to us out of concern for our well being.

By the time I started my residency in family practice at the University of Massachusetts, I had a pretty thorough understanding of NFP. When I was a busy first-year intern, a brave NFP teacher came and spoke to our very anti-NFP residency program. She was trained at the Pope Paul VI Institute in Omaha, where research was being done into the applications of NFP to other areas of women's health. After the presentation, I picked up a brochure from the Institute and almost without thinking, I stuck it into a folder I was keeping with ideas for electives that I might want to take in the coming years.

As the time came to choose my electives, there was a week that I could not fill. I made dozens of phone calls, trying to set up a course. Everything seemed to be either filled to capacity or scheduled at a time I wasn't available. Finally, I pulled out the folder I had kept with ideas for electives and I found the Pope Paul VI Institute brochure. The dates for the program matched the empty space in my schedule exactly. My residency agreed to pay for my flight to Omaha, but the tuition was expensive and Suzanne and I were broke as broke could be. To my surprise the Diocese of Worcester gave me a $1,000 grant, telling me they were sure I'd be able to pay it back in time. When I asked the terms of repayment, the monsignor just smiled and said, "You'll eventually repay it many times over in ways you would not expect."

Attending that elective in Omaha was amazing, just like being up on the yardarm. It changed the course of my career in medicine. After completing my residency I went into practice in Gardner, Massachusetts. I am a family physician and as a result of my experience in Omaha a major component of my practice is NaProTechnology, helping women with infertility and delivering babies.

NaProTech is the child of NFP. Over the past 25 years research done at the Pope Paul VI Institute and elsewhere has led to a detailed understanding of the mechanisms underlying normal fertility, infertility, and female hormone regulation. Like NFP, NaProTech involves charting of cervical mucus, but it goes further to find the root causes of problems such as infertility, premenstrual syndrome, postpartum depression, irregular or abnormal menstrual bleeding and other gynecologic problems. NaProTech focuses on healing the disordered reproductive system when there's some disruption and does so in a way that is consistent with Catholic teaching.

For example, in treatment of postpartum depression we have a 98 percent cure rate with a single shot of progesterone. The patient's symptoms often improve within a half an hour. Once during a lecture I was giving on postpartum depression, a man in the audience stood up to speak. "Oh no, now I'm in trouble. This is probably another doctor who doesn't believe in NaProTech," I thought to myself. But I was wrong. He was a husband who had some encouraging words for my approach to treatment. "My wife had been suffering for three months after our son was born," he said. "She had been on all kinds of treatments. Nothing worked. I brought her all the way from Providence to your office in Gardner. You gave her the progesterone and by the time we got back on Route 2, my wife was a different person! She wasn't so anxious or paranoid. She was making sense again."

In the treatment of infertility NaProTech is radically different from the approach used by most physicians, which centers on the use of In-vitro Fertilization (IVF). NaProTech enables couples to achieve pregnancy naturally. It is not only respectful of a woman's health, but it is also respectful of the dignity of the relationship between husband and wife. And further, it upholds the dignity of the child and the child's right to be conceived through the loving action of a mother and father, not through the work of someone in a lab coat with a Petri dish. Charting the biomarkers of a woman's cycles tells us whether there is sufficient mucus to facilitate the entry of sperm and whether her hormone levels are sufficient to maintain a pregnancy. With IVF, in contrast, a team of scientists conceives life in a Petri dish and subsequently put a few embryos back in the woman's body. IVF treats life as a commodity. NaProTech treats life as a gift.

By fine-tuning the treatment to the specific anomalies of a woman's own cycle, we are able to achieve a far better rate of live births per patient than with IVF. Furthermore, with IVF 6.7 embryos die for every successful birth. And that's just the *implanted* embryos. That figure doesn't include the embryos that are discarded or destroyed through pre-implantation testing. A woman who conceives through NaProTech is 96 percent less likely to miscarry than one who conceives through IVF.

How do we do it? How does NaProTech help with infertility? Sometimes the answer is very simple. I've helped so many women achieve pregnancy just by advising them to stop taking vitamin C because it dries up cervical mucus. Most women take vitamin C to prevent colds but when they stop taking it, they achieve a pregnancy. I may prescribe vitamin B6, which helps the body produce cervical mucus. Or I may give progesterone to make up for the fact that the woman's ovaries aren't producing enough. These simple measures can often solve the problems before I have even met the patient. If not, there are many other medical and surgical treatments that I can employ, all in concert with the teachings of the Church.

Despite that record of success, even Catholic doctors dismiss NaProTech in the treatment of infertility. Without even investigating or treating the underlying causes of infertility, doctors will recommend IVF as the "only way" to treat it. Patients often go through several unsuccessful rounds of IVF, without realizing that there is an alternative treatment method that doesn't involve the conception of embryos in a laboratory.

The Church teaches us to respect life in all of its stages, at its beginning and also at its end. Our faith tells us there are three reasons why persons have value. We are made in the image and likeness of God; we are saved by the suffering, passion and death of Jesus on the Cross; and we are destined for eternal life in heaven. As a family physician, I can help my patients to appreciate their great value and to develop a sense of wonder at how their bodies are designed.

Respect for the body begins when children are five or six years old. I'm not just talking about "sex education." I might say to a child as I'm examining him, "Isn't your body cool? Listen to how your heart pumps your blood." Or I might say, "Your mom's breastfeeding your brother over there. Isn't it cool how God made her body so she can feed the baby?" I try to help children learn to appreciate that the Creator had a hand in how their bodies are designed.

With another child the message might be, "Your body's growing fast. God wants you to be strong and to accomplish important things in the world. But you need to eat those vegetables. They're better for your body than Twinkies." With this approach I am giving them a sense of responsibility for the care of their bodies. As adolescence unfolds, the conversation keeps evolving. "Now you're growing this pubic hair. It isn't something to be embarrassed about; it's a natural ventilation system, because you're going to be sweating more now that you're nearly grown up. Wow, what a wonderful design!" If children have learned to respect their bodies this prepares them for the challenges of adolescence.

I named my medical practice "In His Image" because it helps remind me that each patient is made in God's image. I try to listen to each patient and care for him or her as I would for Christ. I once heard a story about Mother Teresa caring for a dying patient with such a terrible stench and dreadful wounds that it was making another sister physically repulsed. The other sister asked, "Mother, how can you do that?" She answered, "Because I can see through the wounds and the smell. I see Christ."

My approach doesn't mean that I don't sometimes get angry with patients or set limits with them. I also have to be a good steward of my time and resources. Compassion is essential. You have to suffer with the patient, to take on his or her suffering to some degree, if you are going to have any influence on the relationship. We must take the time to listen, to understand what the patient is going through so that the patient feels valued.

One of my patients whom I helped to achieve a pregnancy told me, "I've met a lot of doctors, but you're the first *physician* I've ever met. You cared about my whole being: my marriage relationship, my faith point of view, my illnesses, my nutrition, my family history, and my future health. When a doctor includes the spiritual and emotional along with the physical, and is intent on that person's entire welfare, that's a true physician."

I'm always learning from my patients. Sometimes the lessons are practical such as when a patient recently told me about a support group for mothers of special-needs children. And sometimes the lessons are spiritual. Once I had a patient who had traveled a long way to see me. At the end of the visit she asked if we could pray together. I told her I'd love to but I did not know how. She took my hand and called on the name of the Father, and led us both in prayer. It was a very special moment and taught me a lot about how one might pray with patients.

Trying to practice medicine in an authentically Catholic way does involve swimming against the tide—and sometimes that tide feels like a tsunami! Yet there are many patients who have come to appreciate their Church's teaching and want to approach human sexuality in a godly way. They aren't finding any support in the medical community and often go to great lengths and sometimes travel great distances to find a physician who will be supportive. They tell me, "My doctor doesn't understand my values."

Some doctors tell me, "I'd loved to be involved in NFP, but my teenage patients have multiple boyfriends. You can't expect them to do charts or pay attention to their fertility. So I prescribe contraceptives." Yet this is a disservice to the patient. We shouldn't be facilitating these immoral relationships. We should be teaching them something better, helping them climb out of these relationships. If we don't, these young people are going to be stuck in a destructive cycle for the rest of their lives. Pills and condoms are not the answer.

It is important to be consistent with our advice to teenagers and not give them mixed messages. Some parents tell their teen, "I expect you not to have sex until you're married, but if you do, use a condom." The advice to use a contraceptive defeats the whole message and makes it easier to fail. What we should be saying instead is, "I know it's hard; I know there are urges; I know there are times when it's a challenge. But you can do it; you can stay chaste. I'm holding the bar high for you, and if you're having trouble, come to me and I'd be happy to talk to you about it."

Being a Catholic physician isn't easy but only once in 20 years have I had a patient who dismissed my philosophy completely. It was a very busy day and I was already running behind on my appointments when a 14-year-old girl came in to see me. Her mother was out in the waiting room. It said on the girl's chart that the mom wanted her daughter put on the birth control pill.

I could have said, "I'm sorry, but I don't prescribe the pill." Instead I said, "So how's it going? How's your world?" She told me she had started dating a boy. "That's great!" I said. "We need boyfriends. We need to be able to meet lots of people and talk with them about who we are as persons."

We started talking about fertility and sexuality. She told me, "My mother wants me on the pill. She thinks I'm having sex with this guy, but I'm not."

"Your mother's trying to protect you and this is the only way she knows how to do that," I answered. "You need to help her understand that you're not having sex, that you appreciate how wonderfully your body is made. Can you bring it up and talk with her about it?" She said that she could.

Then I asked her directly if she was interested in taking the pill. "No!" she said. "I don't want to have sex with this guy." "That's great!" I told her. I tried to further empower her by explaining how often relationships fail when couples have sex before marriage. It's like putting the cart before the horse—the horse has a hard time steering that cart and the most important elements of the relationship cannot flourish. I told her that sexual activity before marriage increases the risk of single parenthood and divorce. Of course, this didn't take just a 15-minute appointment time slot; ours was a 35-minute conversation.

Well, once we'd said goodbye and I was with my next patient, I heard a hammering on the exam room door. My receptionist told me that the girl's mother was irate and demanded to talk with me. So now I had the daughter outside in the waiting room and the mother, who was beside herself with anger, in the examination room. "I took time off work and took her out of school, and I paid the co-pay, and you didn't put her on the pill!" she declared. "I want her on the pill. I'm her mother."

I explained that her daughter and I had talked about her wish to protect her daughter, which deflated her anger a little. Then I told her, "I don't prescribe the pill."

"Then what did you waste our time for?" she raged.

"We had a wonderful talk." I told the mother. "You should ask her about it."

"This is ludicrous!" the mother snapped and stormed out. This incident reminded me that as Catholic physicians we must be prepared to experience rejection.

We must also be prepared to be tested. Several years ago I faced a huge challenge. Our society has separated the unitive and procreative aspects of the marital act.[15] This separation has led to all sorts of immoral actions including contraception, IVF, two women trying to have a child, or even a woman having a child using a dead man's sperm. It was in this last issue that I was particularly tested. A patient called me one day, frantic, and said, "Dr. Carpentier, you've got to help me! My son, my only son was just killed in an accident. He just got married a month ago. He was just killed two hours ago! His body was brought to the ER. I want you to help arrange for his sperm to be harvested so I can have a grandson."

How could I say no? And yet, how could I say yes? I was confident in what I needed to say but how would I translate that message to someone in such distress? Finally, I said, "This is going to be hard for you to process, but I don't think it is in your best

---

15. According to Catholic teaching God intends for the marital act (sexual intercourse) to unite couples physically, emotionally and spiritually (its unitive purpose) and at the same time intends it for the producing of children (the procreative purpose). These two purposes of the marital act must not be separated.

interest or in the interest of your future grandchild to be brought into the world this way." She couldn't comprehend my words. "They won't listen to me! I want you to call them and help me," she replied. "I need you to help me harvest the sperm. I can't believe you're talking to me this way." With every bit of compassion I could muster, I replied, "I cannot participate in that. It's not worthy of that child's dignity." She hung up the phone.

So I pray—what else can I do? I ask God to help me.

Being a busy physician I have a special fear. Every day I pray, "Please, God, don't ask me to be in two places at once." I'm always afraid I'll have a lady getting ready to deliver her baby and at the same moment another patient in the ICU crashing. It would break my heart to be unable to care for any of my patients when they are in crisis. So I pray, "Lord, I'll give up going home to supper and work long hours, just don't let two things happen at once." And sure enough, two or three times a week, I'll be working in the hospital or in my office, writing my last note at say 7:30 p.m., with my dinner already getting cold, and my beeper will go off. So I'll say, "Hi, God. Thanks for sending me just one problem at a time."

Sometimes I struggle with the concept of "prayer" because it's a word that's kind of confusing to me. I wouldn't know how to answer if you asked me, "Were you praying up there on the yardarm of the *Westward?*" That's because I see my whole life as a prayer. I look at prayer as an extension of the celebration of the Mass into my daily life, into my family and my relationships with people. Sometimes it's a simple running question, "What would Jesus do with this minute, this day, this interaction with this person or this patient? What should I say to my son? How do I handle this disagreement with my wife?" If you're always asking those questions, then your whole life is a prayer.

We need prayer but we also need endurance. I love soccer and, in fact, I have a t-shirt that says, "Soccer is Life." Even though I'm almost 50 years old, I'm still out on the soccer field every chance I get, coaching and playing. There are times when I get tired and I just want to bend over and rest, but then I see the ball going over to my area on the field and I've got to get over there to cover it. I have to endure, to play my part for the team, just as I did when I was a kid.

Prayer and endurance are important, but as a Catholic physician I've found I also need the support and fellowship of other Catholic physicians. About 12 years ago someone told me about the Catholic Medical Association. I remember going with my wife to the national meeting in Chicago—it was wonderful! The speakers were impressive and there was great fellowship. Since then I've gone to a number of national CMA meetings. As a physician my primary responsibility is to care for my patients, but I also have realized that as a Catholic physician I need to be involved in supporting work at the regional and national levels. About three years ago a group of us here in the Diocese of Worcester started a local guild of the CMA, of which I am currently president. I got involved for my own benefit and so that I could help support other Catholic physicians in our area.

Over the years I've become involved in other ways at the regional and national levels. For many years I've given talks on natural family planning and NaProTech. I gave my first talk after I finished my training at the Pope Paul VI Institute in Omaha. I was still a family practice resident at the time. The presentation was to my fellow residents during our noontime continuing medical education program. It was difficult because my colleagues basically laughed and scoffed at what I had to say. They said, "You don't know what you're talking about." But I've continued giving talks ever since to anyone who would listen—NFP groups, home-schooling moms, Catholic high schools, groups of priests, and others. Last month I gave a talk on NaProTech to the Worcester Guild. About two years ago, I even gave a talk at the Vatican, which was an amazing experience. The Pope's theologian and several cardinals attended.

Back in 1989 I became a member of the American Academy of Fertility Care Professionals. The AAFCP was founded about 25 years ago to foster, advance and promote the Creighton Model FertilityCare System, NaProTechnology and related fields. The Academy maintains a system for credentialing doctors and other professionals who are trained in NaProTech and Creighton Model NFP. I am currently president of the organization even though as a busy family doctor it has been hard to find the time. They had actually been asking me to serve as president for the past five years, but I felt I couldn't accept because of my work and family commit-ments. Finally, this last year with my wife's approval, I decided to go ahead and accept the position.

My work with the Academy, giving talks on NFP and NaProTech, and work with the Catholic Medical Association and Worcester Guild are really important to me. I see this work as helping our culture to survive. It seems to be spiraling downward. I picture the culture like an ocean filled with sharks that are destroying people—a culture of death. But the Church is like an island of safety where life is respected, where chastity is valued, where marriage is upheld, where fertility is welcomed. I try to do what I can to help others get onto that island.

As I get older and more experienced with the ways in which God works in the world, I'm able to look back at my life and say, "Wow, look how He let those desires and interests and natural inclinations work." God used my love of seeing Jacques Cousteau, with his power scooters underwater in the coral reefs, to motivate me to study hard and do well in my science courses. Then He said, "Um, I've got a switch for you. What would you think about being a doctor?" When I was six years old, He didn't say, "How would you feel about doing NaProTechnology?" If He had, I would have said, "Are you nuts? I'd rather be scuba diving."

But when I was out at sea on the *Westward* studying marine biology God suggested, "I think you'd enjoy a career helping people." He didn't tell me that I'd meet a chaplain in med school who would point me toward NFP. Or that three years later, I'd be at a luncheon and someone would give me a brochure on NaProTech, which would become my life's passion.

Looking back, I can see that my life has been a series of small "yeses" to God's call. Do you know it's God calling? Not always. It's not like the Angel Gabriel in all his glory is in front of you saying, "Do you want to be a doctor?" Instead it's little tiny steps. Sure, I'll go to that conference. Yes, I'll talk to that chaplain. God uses our aspirations and desires to help us accomplish His mission.

In my life, God's calling has been gentle, not overwhelming as it was for Mary at the Annunciation. To me God said, "You can say yes or no. If you say no, maybe I'll come back later and give you another chance." And sometimes when that next opportunity comes, you realize, "Hmmm. I said no, and look what happened. Maybe I should have said yes the first time."

Suzanne and I have been blessed with four sons—four young men. It's been amazing to watch them develop. All four are passionate about giving back to the community, like me and my dad, but each in different ways. One wants to be a gym teacher to keep kids healthy; another wants to be a history teacher; one wants to be a lawyer to fight for authentic health care reform; and one is working on solar power to save our environment. Currently none of them wants to be a doctor! Could I pressure them to go in that direction? Maybe, but my way is not God's way. God is still working in their lives, calling them as He called me.

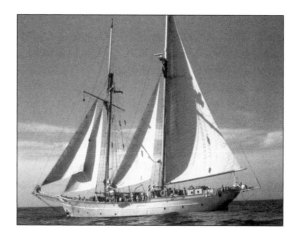

The Westward

— Ad Majorem Dei Gloriam —

5

Dr. E. Joanne Angelo

THY OWN SOUL A SWORD SHALL PIERCE

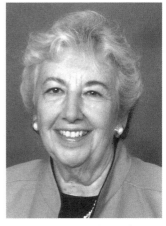

Both medicine and the Catholic faith run in my family. My grandparents came from Italy and settled in Boston's North End, bringing their Catholic tradition with them. Both my parents were physicians. My mother graduated from Tufts Medical School in 1928; my dad graduated the year before. So I came to be a doctor very naturally.

My parents married as young physicians during the Great Depression and like many people at that time they did whatever work was available. They took calls on nights and weekends; my dad took care of prisoners and my mother did home deliveries. Later on, they were able to specialize by serving apprenticeships— that was the training system back then. My mother became an allergist and my father a surgeon with a specialty in proctology.

My mother continued to practice medicine while I was growing up. Once when I was an undergraduate at Mount Holyoke College, a classmate said to me, "Your mother's a doctor? Didn't you ever feel neglected?" I thought, "Neglected?" I'd never even considered that. For one thing, my mother only worked part-time, and my grandmother was always home to take care of my sister and me. I even came home from school for lunch every day and she would have a hot meal prepared for us.

But it wasn't always easy. I remember waking up one night when I was seven years old and hearing my baby sister crying. She didn't stop, so I got up and went to see what was wrong. My mother wasn't there and my father was trying, unsuccessfully, to quiet the baby. I asked him, "Where's Mummy?" He told me she had to go out to take care of a woman who was having a baby. Not long after that my mother switched her practice and became an allergist so that she wouldn't have to go out at night anymore.

During my childhood, my mother and father shared an office, and my sister and I used to go to spend time there on our school vacations. My mother would take me to her allergy clinic at the hospital and the nurses there would amuse me while I watched the patients going in and out of my mother's office. If we were driving on a long trip in the winter, when it was cold, my mother would say to me, "Please help me put on my gloves. This is how you hold the gloves in the operating room." And she'd have me hold them the way they did in surgery. So I guess in many ways, we were brought up with a medical model.

In our family, as in many other Italian families back then, it was the women who went to church regularly. I went with my mother, my sister and my maternal grandmother, who lived with us. In typical fashion, my dad didn't come to Mass, although he had a very deep faith. Before they were married, my parents had moved from the North End. My younger sister and I grew up in Cambridge. None of us attended parochial school—I went to public schools through middle school, then attended a private high school. The faith we experienced was a cultural faith. We lived our faith in our daily lives.

I did participate in the religious education program at our parish and attended Sunday school. I had to be prepared for Confirmation by the priest at the rectory, because my long school days did not permit me to attend classes with the other candidates. At one point I won some sort of prize for an exam and since I couldn't be there to pick it up, I had to go to the convent on a Saturday to get it. I'd never been inside a convent before. Once inside I saw all the young nuns cleaning and having a great time. Until then I had no idea that they were human beings and had fun, just like my friends and me.

But some childhood faith experiences impressed themselves deeply on my mind. I can remember walking with my grandmother in the winter, when it was cold and dark, to early morning Mass on a holy day. And I can remember visiting my other grandparents, the Sicilian part of the family. That grandmother had a little altar in her room and pictures of the saints all around. I would occasionally stay with them for a weekend and whenever we went out to shop or to do anything else, my grandmother would say, "There's nothing more important to do than to visit Our Lord." So before we went anywhere else, we always stopped in at church to make a visit to the Blessed Sacrament.

Later in his life, my dad decided he would go to Mass with us. I don't know what prompted him to do that, but he told us, "You girls look so nice, you need an escort."

My father died fairly young, at 65. He had a heart attack while he was at a medical meeting in Bermuda with my mother. There were lots of doctors around to respond when he became ill. He was taken to a local hospital where, amazingly, there was a Canadian chaplain who happened to be of Sicilian descent, like my dad. He went into Dad's room to talk with him and when he came out, he told us, "He's a man of very great faith." In his heart, Dad had always been faith filled and he returned to the Sacraments just before he died.

At Mount Holyoke College there was no Catholic chaplain, Catholic club, or Newman Center.[16] The administration apparently felt we didn't need it, because our college was supposed to be a "fellowship of faiths." But not long after I started my studies there, a polio epidemic broke out, and we were quarantined on campus. That meant we couldn't leave to attend Mass. So we Catholic students found each other and began to gather on Sundays to pray the rosary together. We realized that we needed help to support and nurture our faith. We weren't getting it.

So we reached out to the Newman Clubs at the nearby University of Massachusetts, Smith College and Amherst College. The chaplains there helped us to found the Newman Club of South Hadley—it wasn't called the Newman Club of Mount Holyoke, because the college wouldn't endorse it. Now we had access not only to Mass, but also to other resources to help build our faith. We had seminars on Catholic thought and theology with the chaplains and we established a reserved reading shelf of Catholic authors in our library.

At that time, I wasn't convinced that I wanted to be a doctor although I did know I wanted to work with children. I studied psychology at Mount Holyoke and although I enjoyed the subject matter, I didn't like the department very much. So I transferred into early childhood education, but I couldn't quite see myself in a classroom. Finally, because I wanted to work with children and liked psychology, I decided to be a child psychiatrist.

However, I was very much afraid that studying psychiatry would cost me my faith. At that time, there was a real animosity

---

16. Named in honor of John Henry Cardinal Newman, the Newman Centers are centers for Catholic students at many non-Catholic universities throughout the world.

toward religion in the field of psychiatry. Today, that attitude is pretty much a thing of the past because psychiatrists are looking more carefully at the spiritual elements of their patients' lives. But when I was a student, the prevailing attitude toward religion was dismissive. I think that came from the psychoanalytic tradition of Freud, which didn't recognize the value of a transcendental faith. It was almost as if Freud had a microscope hyper-focused on the sexual elements of the human person, and didn't see the rest—the elements of love, maturity and spirituality, which Pope John Paul II in his writings so eloquently integrated for us.

When classes ended one spring I attended a weeklong seminar, taught by a Dominican priest, at Our Lady of the Elms College in Chicopee, Massachusetts. The sharp focus on Catholic philosophy and theology led me to think that I wasn't equipped to be a psychiatrist. When I made my first retreat, I spoke to the retreat master about my concerns. He said, "Oh, if God wants you to be a psychiatrist, He'll pour into you the graces you need." But I wasn't sure how that was going to happen.

I was still uncertain about going into psychiatry when I reached medical school. I went to Tufts, my parents' alma mater. In a class of 116 students, only four were women. Some of us were Catholic, but at Tufts like Mount Holyoke, we didn't have many Catholic resources or much support. We had two "borrowed" chaplains from Brandeis and MIT, who offered us case studies in ethics and other courses on the side. Several of the male students at Tufts had been to Catholic colleges in the area, but they had no use for psychiatry and they wouldn't even attend the psych lectures. That certainly didn't help me very much. But I held on to the encouraging words from the retreat master, "If God wants you to be a psychiatrist, He'll pour into you the graces you need." Then, later that year at Christmas Midnight Mass, I saw one of our lecturers, a psychoanalyst whom I liked very much, going up to receive Communion. I thought, "If she can do it, I can do it!"

In my third year of med school, I met a group of women who were opening a student residence called Bayridge—it's right next door to my present office. Bayridge was run by members of Opus Dei, an organization within the Catholic Church that helps people live Christian lives in the middle of the world. I visited the residence during my junior year, and in my senior year, I moved in.

Life at Bayridge was wonderful, because we had Mass every day in our own chapel. Our residence was home to an international group of about 30 women, both graduate and undergraduate students. I was the only one studying medicine, but there were many other professions represented. There I was able to take courses in philosophy and theology, which strengthened me spiritually. And there I found encouragement to go forward into psychiatry.

Sometimes I really needed that encouragement. I remember in one of my psychiatry classes in med school, the professor was going on and on about how religion is a crutch, something only required by neurotics. Well, at the time I happened to be reading the writings of St. Theresa of Avila, and I thought, "Hmmm…*she's* not neurotic." I read how she distinguished between the nuns in her community who were truly pious and those who were anorexic or had other psychological issues. So I brought my professor a chapter from the book to read. And at the next class he said, "Well, there's one exception to the rule that religion is for neurotics, and that's St. Theresa of Avila."

Maybe bringing up such a contradiction to a professor was a bold move, but the faculty of the psychiatry department grew to like me. Psychiatry was one of the few fields where women were welcome. We were told, "We're so glad to have you. These psychiatric patients want to talk to a woman." The same was true in pediatrics where we were told, "We're glad to have you—the children relate well to women." So, perhaps it's not surprising that I went into child psychiatry (which had been my goal all along). I could see that if children were troubled at an early age and not helped, their lives could be destroyed. I particularly wanted to help children who were suffering from what I was calling childhood depression. It wasn't accepted as a diagnosis then, though of course it is now. But I could see that these children were sad. I could see that they had learning disabilities, that they were traumatized. I wanted to use my professional skills to reach out to them and help them and their families.

My desire to help children led me into a pediatric psychiatry internship at Boston City Hospital. City Hospital served the poorest of the poor; people who couldn't get treated anywhere else in Boston came to us. I saw a lot of very sick babies and children. But there was also a lot of faith there. There were many immigrant families from Puerto Rico who had a strong Catholic faith and there was a Jesuit parish right across the street, which served the hospital and nursing school.

During my internship, I diagnosed a child with leukemia only to see him die just a month later. He was really suffering and he didn't like his intravenous infusions. I'd tell him, "Come on, David, just offer it up." It got to where he'd see me coming into his room with a syringe and he would try to smile and say, "Okay, Dr. Angelo, I'll offer it up!" His parents were so distressed they couldn't bear to be with him so I, as a young intern, decided I needed to stay with David on his last night. My resident insisted that I go home and get some sleep, but I refused to leave him. As I watched over him, he was delirious but nonetheless, he seemed to be having a conversation with someone. "My name is David…I'll be 10 years old in a couple of days," he said. "I play baseball. But you can't play baseball before the ground thaws. No, I think I'll wait till tomorrow. Tomorrow's Sunday. I think my mom and dad will come after they go to church."

As it turned out, the next day *was* a Sunday and his parents *did* come and he died with both of them at his bedside. Because of the bond that had built up between us, I went to his funeral. At the cemetery, the ground was just thawing as they buried him on his 10th birthday. That incident made a great impression on me.

I know my faith must have been tested while I was in training, but I seem to have suppressed those memories. I do recall situations in which I was seeing pregnant adolescent girls who were considering abortion. In those days before it was fully legalized, an abortion required a letter from a psychiatrist stating that the abortion was required because the patient had mental health problems. In my early training, I was asked to do these evaluations, but I never found a reason to order the abortion. It wasn't because I was taking a pro-life stance. I was just working on a case-by-case basis. But I was criticized for that. Actually, the current thinking, even in the pro-abortion community, is that psychiatric illness may be a contraindication for abortion, because the aftereffects can be worse for these patients.

After my internship I went on to train in adult psychiatry at Boston State Hospital—3,000 patients, who were there for life. That was a very trying two years. We rotated through the admissions unit, then to a unit where patients stayed for a year of treatment. If they didn't get well, they went to the hospital's East Side, which might as well have been in Siberia because they never got out of there. This was in the early 1960s, when we psychiatrists were using a lot of shock treatment and had just stopped using sedative tubs to treat patients. Sedative tubs involved immersing patients into tubs of warm water with a tarp covering all but their heads. The first anti-psychotic medications had become available but those turned patients into zombies. Thankfully, today we have much better medications and treatment methods available for patients.

At Boston State Hospital I learned that even patients with very serious mental illness could have great faith. I remember one psychotic woman who was in a quiet room—what's often called a "padded room"—who was saying aspirations, like "Jesus, Mary and Joseph; Jesus, Mary and Joseph; Jesus, Mary and Joseph," over and over again. There were two chaplains at the hospital, and they offered Mass regularly for the patients. One would distribute Communion while the other stood behind the patients as they knelt, giving a signal "yes" or "no," depending on whether he judged a person fit to receive Communion because of their mental state that day.

I prayed a lot while I was at Boston State, especially when I was on night duty. I was the only psychiatrist (and still just a resident) in charge of 3,000 patients as well as any new admissions that might come in. And like Boston City Hospital, this was a place that served the poorest of the poor. I rarely was able to sleep. If I got to bed at all in the on-call room, in between phone calls, I would just pray.

After Boston State Hospital, I began training in child psychiatry in community settings and outpatient clinics. I spent a year working with autistic preschoolers, then another working at the child guidance center at Catholic University of America in Washington, D.C. I had some very interesting experiences with the children at the center. For example, I recall one little seven-year-old boy who seemed to have a hard time telling me what was wrong. Finally, after some persistent but gentle prodding, it came out. "I'm in the St. Jude reading group at school," he told me. St. Jude is the patron saint of hopeless cases. He knew that and it made him very, very sad. We needed to sort it all out. He was *depressed*, but he didn't need anti-depressant medication as much as he needed a better way to learn reading … and a change in the name of that reading group!

My work with children in my psychiatric practice here in Boston taught me a lot too. One boy came in to see me the day after the Challenger space shuttle disaster, in which the crew was killed in an explosion just after lift-off. The boy, who was perhaps eight years old, attended a Catholic school, and had been referred to me for violent behavior. As we talked, he told me how he and the other children at school had watched the launch. There was a teacher, Christa MacAuliffe, on board. This boy's mother was a teacher, as well as a single parent. She had told her son before the launch that her dream was to go up in the space shuttle some day. I knew that witnessing the disaster must have been devastating for him.

When I asked him what it was like, watching the launch, and he said, "Oh, people said it was beautiful. But it was terrible! They all died."

Then he paused, so I asked him, "What do you think happens to people when they die?"

He said. "I don't know. What do you think?"

I said, "I asked you first."

He said, "I asked you second!"

I finally gave in. "I think they go to heaven."

"Yeah, but not everybody," he said. "Adam and Eve didn't go to heaven, because they ate that apple. And if they didn't eat that apple, all those bad things wouldn't happen. When I grow up, I'm going to build a time machine so I can go back in time. And I'm going to kill Adam and Eve!"

I was amazed listening to this child. We had a lot of work to do. He had to make sense out of the space shuttle experience somehow, to put the blame somewhere, and to work on the underlying issue, which was his fear of losing his mother, his only parent. But as has happened so many times in my life, I learned more from this young child than I was able to give or teach him.

Another patient of mine was a 12-year-old boy who was depressed because he was moving to another state and was worried about leaving his friends and going to a new school. Also his parents were divorced, and the move would make it harder to visit his father.

"Dr. Angelo," he told me, "there's something else too. Before we leave, my mother is getting married, and I have to give her away to my other mother. What am I going to do on parent-teacher night? Who am I going to bring?" At first I didn't understand and then realized that his mother was marrying another woman. This was very hard for him. There wasn't too much I could do, since they were moving, but I let him talk it out. I encouraged him to spend as much time with his father as he could before he left and to remember that he could visit his father on vacations.

How does a psychiatrist absorb that kind of pain all day? That's where faith comes in. In order to deal with sorrow and suffering, I think that we need someone to lean on. We need to be able to lean on the Lord, to have supportive people around and to maintain a prayer life. I recently gave a talk on suffering from a psychiatric perspective and I mentioned that psychiatrists suffer too, through vicarious traumatization. While I was preparing that talk, I was meditating on the mysteries of the rosary, particularly on the presentation of Jesus in the temple, when Simeon tells Mary, "And thy own soul a sword shall pierce, that, out of many hearts, thoughts may be revealed."[17] And I realized that's the role of the psychiatrist.

Shortly after I gave that talk, we heard news of a tragedy at Fort Hood, where a military psychiatrist went on a rampage and shot a number of people. One of the young soldiers interviewed there said of the shooter, "He heard so many terrible stories for so many years, I think it finally got to him." Imagine.

I go to Mary a lot for help in my role as a psychiatrist. She had to witness her Son's suffering and she couldn't do anything to stop it. But she supported Him and remained a faithful witness, and she co-redeemed humanity as a result. I keep a statue of her here in my office.

When I began my private practice, I didn't advertise myself as a Catholic psychiatrist, partly because I wanted to be open and available to people of all faiths, with all types of problems. That included those who were considering an abortion. I didn't want them to write me off before even coming to talk to me.

About 25 years ago, when the Archdiocese of Boston appointed a new pro-life director, I visited her in her office, which was in my hospital. This was our first pro-life director who wasn't a priest—she was a social worker. I went by to welcome her and tell her that if there was anything I could do, to let me know. Well, you don't say that to a pro-life director unless you *mean* it. She told me, "Well, as a matter of fact, we're starting a new program in the archdiocese called Project Rachel. It's meant to welcome back women after an abortion, to offer them a chance to talk to a priest who understands their issues, to receive the Sacrament of Reconciliation, and also to offer them professional counseling. We have a training

---

17. Luke 2:35 (Douay-Rheims Bible)

session for priests coming up. Have you ever seen anyone in your practice who's had an abortion?" When I told her I had, she invited me to come to the training session and anonymously to share some of my experiences.

One hundred priests, who'd been chosen for this ministry, were at the session. I spoke on the panel just after a woman who had had an abortion. She told the assembly that she had been ready to commit suicide after the abortion, but that she had had an encounter with a priest who offered her hope and a chance for forgiveness. That encounter at the right moment probably saved her life. As she told her story, to my astonishment, a hundred priests wept.

I too was so moved by her story. That was an important moment in my understanding of how I could perhaps help women who had had abortions be reconciled with the Church, and it launched a whole series of events that led to the establishment of Project Rachel in our diocese. Over time I was called on to speak with priests and other diocesan staff members, and eventually I helped start Project Rachel in other dioceses as well. I began to be known publicly as a Catholic psychiatrist.

So many of the post-abortion patients I saw felt that they had committed an unforgivable sin. Some of them had even gone to healing services but they didn't feel better. They saw their failure to be healed as evidence that they'd never be forgiven. There was a real need to introduce them to God's love through priests who could help them, or through other women who had also had abortions and felt as they did. Over time, they understood God's love and forgiveness, and the fact that one day they would be reunited with their children. Pope John Paul II had some beautiful words for them about that hope.[18] As a result, some of them developed a stronger faith, perhaps stronger than anyone else I knew, including myself.

Another pivotal experience for me was standing watch over a good friend who was quite ill with multiple sclerosis that had affected her brain. She was in the ICU on the neurology service.

---

18. "I would like to say a special word to *women who have had an abortion*...Do not give in to discouragement and do not lose hope. Try rather to understand what happened and face it honestly. If you have not already done so, give yourselves over with humility and trust to repentance. The Father of mercies is ready to give you his forgiveness and peace in the Sacrament of Reconciliation. You will come to understand that nothing is definitively lost and you will also be able to ask forgiveness from your child, who is now living in the Lord." Pope John Paul II, encyclical. (*Evangelium Vitae*); 99:1995

My friends and I were with her in shifts, 24 hours a day. She survived and actually lived for 10 years in a kind of locked-in state, barely able to communicate.[19] When she was in the ICU, the chief of neurology asked me if I was interested in participating in a new home-based hospice program that the archdiocese was starting. I told him, "I'm a child psychiatrist. You don't want me." He answered, "Yes, I've seen you at the bedside. We do want you."

So I became a staff member in the department of psychiatry at St. Elizabeth's Medical Center, and I helped found the Good Samaritan Hospice. I worked there for a number of years, making home visits, attending team meetings, and doing a lot of public speaking about hospice as an alternative to physician-assisted suicide. Being at the bedside of dying patients, often along with a priest, was very moving for me, as well as for the priests and families. For one reason or another, many of these families had been alienated from their parishes, but when the priest came to attend to their loved ones in their last illnesses, he would become almost part of the family.

I knew a cancer nurse who was herself dying of cancer. I took some volunteers who were learning about hospice to see her and she told them, "When you have cancer, you have time,"—time for unfinished business. This was certainly true for her. Her son was traveling in Europe and they hadn't been able to find him. But he finally returned and spent some quality time with his mother before she died. As a cancer nurse she had always been teaching, and now her own cancer gave her some time to teach about the illness, about life and death.

I've learned a lot from another woman, a patient of mine, who has a chronic illness and was expected to die within three years of her diagnosis. Yet she's still alive, 15 years later. She once told me that living with a terminal illness is like living on the edge of a cliff, and that Jesus brings us there to help us appreciate how we depend entirely on Him. "It's not easy living on the edge of a cliff," she told me. "It's scary to peer over the edge. Others can even get nervous seeing us so close to the edge that they back away from us. But once we learn that there is nothing to fear when Jesus holds us, then being a 'cliff dweller' can actually make us much stronger and better acquainted with the mystery of life."

She has personally witnessed people backing away from her. But others reached out to her. The first time she showed up at her

---

19. Locked-in state or syndrome is a condition in which the patient is conscious and awake, but cannot move or communicate due to paralysis of the voluntary muscles.

church with a "breathing tube," she had people who'd never spoken to her before come up to ask if they could help her with her heavy oxygen tank. Others told her about relatives or friends who used portable oxygen. This patient has taught me a great deal, and I hope she will continue to do so for a good while. If she's no longer able to come to see me, I will feel privileged if she allows me to visit her and help her through the terminal phase of her illness, whenever that comes.

As a result of my work in hospice psychiatry, I was invited to participate in a conference at the first modern hospice, St. Christopher's in London. While there I met the founder, Dr. Cicily Saunders, a devout Anglican. She took a liking to me, I think because we shared the Christian faith. She took me to meet some of the patients, which she seldom does with visitors. During the conference I discovered that many hospice psychiatrists talk about God all the time. Most physicians have been trained not to talk about God. But when staff members at St. Christopher's gave a case history of a dying patient, they almost always talked about the patient's faith and his or her understanding of God. This was very instructive for me.

I'd always been personally faithful and prayerful, but my work in the fields of post-abortion healing and hospice care gradually made it easier for me to talk with patients about God and religion. I try to ask leading questions, but not to impose my views or my religion on them. And I've learned to make it easier for them to bring it up. The statue of Our Lady in my office isn't in full view of patients, but if they look around, they'll see it. When I ask patients about their school years, they'll usually tell me if they went to Catholic school, and I ask about any church involvement in their family when they were growing up. If it's an elderly patient, they may be more eager to talk about what happens after death and what unfinished business needs to be resolved.

Some people attribute their problems to their religious upbringing. I share the waiting room of my office with a group of psychologists and one of them once came and told me, "You've *got* to change your schedule. There are two nuns sitting out there, waiting to see you, every week at the *same* time I see a patient who was abused by nuns." We worked it out and my colleague arranged for her patient to come on another day. We're all subject to original sin, including nuns, priests and bishops. We need to have mercy and forgive, and at the same time, we need to stop the abuse. I realize we're all flawed and when I hear of such things, I think, "There but for the grace of God go I." Psychosis can hit anyone and often the perpetrators of abuse were victims of abuse themselves when they were young. I'm not trying to excuse abuse or to say we can allow it to happen, but to understand it better so that we can identify it, treat the victims and the perpetrators, and ultimately prevent it.

Part of my quest when I originally went into child psychiatry was to try to help my young patients avert these lifelong problems and, if possible, to solve them within the family. So I still write and speak and work with children and their families.

I look to Viktor Frankl a lot, to his writings on the search for a higher, spiritual meaning in whatever situation is presented to us in life. Alone of all his family, he survived the concentration camps in World War II. I was present at a lecture he gave in 1981 titled, "Man's Search for Ultimate Meaning," which was published in a book by the same name.[20] Dr. Frankl talked about life presenting situations to us as though they were frames in a movie. We have to find meaning in each individual picture as we go along, but we won't know the ultimate meaning until the last frame is shown. A lot of psychiatry now has shifted to a much broader view of the person, integrating the spiritual element, the psyche, soma and spirit. I applaud that.

I go to Mass every day, and I try to pray for a half hour each morning and evening to ask for the grace to care for the people who come to me. That helps me put everything in perspective. I also pray the rosary and do a little spiritual reading and I try to keep up with the encyclicals and other writings of the Pope. The writings of Pope John Paul II have helped me tremendously. I also attend a Catholic retreat every year and, through Opus Dei, I have had the wonderful opportunity to take courses in theology and philosophy, with updates on current Church teaching. And I have a regular confessor, someone to help me so I'm not alone in all of this.

I haven't found very many supportive colleagues in my field. I once was asked to give a talk at the annual meeting of the American Psychiatric Association as part of a panel discussion on whether abortion has negative effects. This talk wasn't scheduled at the main conference site, but down the street and in the basement of another hotel, with no signs directing people. Speakers at the other presentations I attended during the conference were all in favor of abortion. It was very discouraging.

---

20. Victor Frankl. *Man's Search for Ultimate Meaning*. New York: Basic Books, 1997.

But in the registration area of the conference were TV sets, which were showing a film of an audience with Pope John Paul II attended by Dr. Joseph English, who was the APA president at that time, and other international psychiatric leaders. The Pope was giving a beautiful talk about the importance of the psychiatrist's role in treating mentally ill patients. The film loop kept repeating and when I needed to, I'd go out and watch and listen to what the Holy Father was telling us. I was so grateful to Dr. English—for his courage in showing that film to that audience at that time.

At one point during the conference I was so disturbed by the content of the presentations that I felt I needed to go and pray to Our Lady. It took some doing, but I found the cathedral in that city, and after some searching around inside, I found an image of Our Lady of Guadalupe. And there was an inscription of her words to Juan Diego: "Do not be troubled nor disturbed by anything; do not fear illness nor any other distressing occurrence, nor pain. Am I not your mother? Am I not life and health? Have I not placed you on my lap and made you my responsibility? Do you need anything else?" So I went back to the conference, encouraged that she would help me, that she would take me in her lap and wrap her mantle around me, and that I could go ahead with the talk. So I did, even though nobody came except our friends, but it remained on the program and it was officially in the American Psychiatric Association conference record.

After I spoke out publicly about my pro-life position, I remember being heckled when I gave talks. Being heckled is an awful thing, but I remember when I spoke at one women's conference where a group of women in the front row hissed and booed and spit at me. It was very difficult to deal with.

I was once asked to give a talk to the Wellesley College psychology department, by a student from the college who was helping me with research. She invited me to speak to the 10 or 12 members of the college's psychology club in one of the labs on the topic of post-abortion problems in women. I said I would. When I got there, however, I found that the talk had been advertised campus-wide via a notice that simply said, "Psychiatrist to speak on abortion." As a result, I had a huge crowd, taking up all the available chairs, sitting on lab benches, sitting on the floor and lining the walls. I knew most of them were hostile to my viewpoint. After all, what psychiatrist would dare to speak at Wellesley College and say that there was anything wrong with abortion?

During the presentation, I did what I often do, and that was to give case examples and tell stories of women I knew or women I had read about who were deeply troubled after having abortions. As I spoke, I could see the students' hostility melt. One young woman, who had been sitting cross-legged on the top of a lab desk, slipped down into a chair and then gradually slid practically down under the table. You could see that she was very moved by what I was saying. I spoke to them about the faith journeys of many of these women. One girl asked me, "If you don't believe in anything, how can you ever deal with this?" So I talked about Victor Frankl and his thoughts on finding meaning in whatever situation life presents you. I played a recording of a folk song written by a woman who had had an abortion. She sang about her child, whom she had named Zephyr. He had been a storm in her life but, as she came to terms with her abortion, he became a gentle breeze. I could see that the story really got to my audience. Personal stories touch hearts and that's the way I like to teach about this issue.

A young faculty member, who had come into the lab during my talk, sat down in the back with a stack of blue books to correct. Afterwards he came up to me and told me, "I got so involved in what you were saying that I didn't correct any of these exams. Students come up to my office to talk to me during office hours, but it's not always class they want to talk about. If they're having trouble dealing with issues like this, where can I send them?"

It's been hard to discover colleagues in the Faith, so the Catholic Medical Association has been a wonderful thing for me. Being with other members helps me feel very much at home and supported. Founded in 1912, our guild here in Boston is the oldest in the country. The CMA has local guilds in many parts of the U.S. Because we have national meetings, I now can identify other Catholic psychiatrists and other physicians of like mind. We reach out and help medical students and young doctors. My own experience has made me realize how important it is to reach out to young people because in medical school, I didn't know how I'd survive in the faith if I went into psychiatry. Seeing one of my teachers at the Christmas Midnight Mass while I was a medical student at Tufts really encouraged me. So I hope my story and the others in this book will help people who want to go into medicine to understand that the profession doesn't have to weaken your faith, and, in fact, that practicing medicine can actually make it stronger.

A number of years ago, I worked with Dr. Joseph Stanton[21] here in Boston to develop an updated version of the Hippocratic Oath.[22] At most U.S. medical schools, students no longer take the traditional oath at graduation. Dr. Stanton wanted to reinstate the principles of the original oath, updating the language to include doctors of both genders, and to address support for life from conception to natural death. I was part of a large group that worked on re-writing the oath and was one of several people who gave talks about the revised version to make it more widely known. The oath has been translated into many different languages and it's been a real help in bringing medical students to the full realization of what it means to be a doctor. One medical school in Spain, where they hadn't taken the Hippocratic Oath in 50 years, got hold of it, translated it into Spanish and began to use it. In many places the Catholic Medical Association has a special dinner with members and med school graduates, at which the graduates can take the oath together with those who are renewing it. The whole process has turned out to be a wonderful thing.

Another thing that has enriched my faith life in my practice has been the Pontifical Academy for Life. Pope John Paul II founded it in 1994 around the time he promulgated *Evangelium Vitae* (*The Gospel of Life*), to help people put his pro-life teachings into practice around the world. The Academy is also a forum for international experts in fields related to pro-life issues to share research and updates from their countries. About 13 years ago, I was appointed to the Academy as a corresponding member. We hold annual meetings in Rome that each year are focused on a particular topic such as end-of-life issues, early embryology, legal or political questions, philosophy, and theology as they apply to pro-life issues.

It's been a wonderful experience to meet pro-life leaders from around the world. Our meetings resemble the Tower of Babel because we're all speaking different languages, although simultaneous translations are provided at the large, general meetings. Nevertheless it helps to know more than one language, because the conversations at meals and during coffee breaks are really the heart of the sessions. The annual meetings provide me with a wonderful opportunity to be among like-minded people of deep faith from all over the world. I've had the

---

21. Dr. Joseph R. Stanton (1927-1997)

22. The full text of the restatement of the Hippocratic Oath can be found at: http://www.worcestercma.org/Hippocratic.html.

opportunity to speak several times before the Academy, on end-of-life issues, the hospice movement, and on post-abortion reconciliation and healing. I've also reported on the U.S. Conference of Catholic Bishops' millennial multimedia campaign (which reached out to women and men who had suffered the tragedy of abortion) and on the pro-life teachings of St. Josemaria Escriva, the founder of Opus Dei.

The first pro-life article I ever had published was in the Catholic Medical Association's journal, *The Linacre Quarterly.* It was a piece about how abortion negatively affects women.[23] Because of the article, I received the quarterly's annual award for excellence in medical and moral journalism—I who had not done well in high school or college English! That paper took on a life of its own. I was asked to condense it for the newsletter of the National Catholic Bioethics Center and then the Human Life Review asked to re-publish the condensed version.

Then I got a call from an editor at Dushkin-McGraw Hill asking if I would allow my piece to be included in a book titled *Taking Sides: Clashing Views on Controversial Issues in Abnormal Psychology.*[24] The book was to be in a point-counterpoint format, dealing with a range of issues including schizophrenia, ADHD, pornography and violence on television. My piece would address the question: Does abortion have negative effects on women? At first I was very hesitant about giving permission to include the article because I wasn't sure what the other view would be and, what's more, the editor wouldn't tell me. But after talking to a friend who had done a piece for this series, I agreed to allow them to re-publish the article. As it turned out, the opposing view was written by a pro-abortion activist who had no academic credentials. Sometime after the book came out, I spoke to a pro-life group at Boston College. Several nursing students came up and one told me, "We just read your paper in our nursing psychology class." The fact that this piece is still being quoted in different publications, is still being taught in classes, and still has an effect on readers has encouraged me a lot in my writing and speaking.

In my travels, I have been privileged to meet the two most recent Popes. I was invited to meet Pope Benedict XVI at an international meeting on post-abortion and post-divorce issues for

23. E. Joanne Angelo, "Psychiatric Sequelae of Abortion: The Many Faces of Post-Abortion Grief," Linacre Quarterly 59:69-80, May 1992.
24. Halgin, Richard P. *Taking Sides: Clashing Views in Abnormal Psychology.* Columbus: McGraw-Hill/Dushkin, 2000.

children and families at the Lateran University in Rome. Since I was an invited speaker, I was also invited to attend the papal audience and was presented to the Pope personally. It was really a great thrill. I had a number of chances to meet Pope John Paul II through the Pontifical Academy of Life's annual meetings, which typically included an audience with the Holy Father. John Paul always addressed the group and, as long as his health permitted, tried to greet everyone. I was there in his last year, when he was too frail to even go to the window for the Angelus.[25] They filmed him at his desk, giving the Angelus talk, but he couldn't speak. It was clearly so frustrating for him and we lived through that suffering with him.

But I remember one papal audience with Pope John Paul II long before that, when his health was better. When I went up to kneel individually before him, I told him I was a psychiatrist from Boston, working with post-abortion women, and also a member of Opus Dei. "We love you very much. We pray for you every day," I told him. And he put his hand on my cheek and he said, "God bless you. God bless you." It was such a wonderful blessing that afterwards I felt as though I could fly home without a plane. And now, when he becomes a saint, I can consider myself a relic!

When you're in Vatican City in St. Peter's Basilica, the sense that the Church is universal in time and space becomes very real. I've been in Rome several times for the feast of the Chair of St. Peter. There's a statue of St. Peter seated in his chair as you enter the Basilica and on that day, he's clothed in red vestments and wears the Papal triple tiara. On that day there are also flowers, candles and special vespers for the current Pope. When you experience that feast in Rome, it's like St. Peter is really present. You can go down beneath the altar into the crypt that holds his actual bones. To see them, and then to see the current Holy Father, brings home the universality and timelessness of the Church and is truly a wonderful experience. But the wonder of a visit there is not limited to the Basilica. I also love to watch the children from all parts of the world—Italy, America, Asia, Europe—who are always chasing pigeons in St. Peter's Square. At St. Peter's you truly experience the Church Universal.

Spurred on by Pope John Paul II, I frequently return to the parable of the Good Samaritan in my own prayer. John Paul

---

25. Since Pope John XXIII in the 1960s, the popes have broadcast an address on Sundays at noon. The speech ends with the Pope reciting the Angelus, a traditional prayer that is recited in many churches, monasteries, and convents three times daily, at 6:00 a.m., noon, and 6:00 p.m.

explained that the suffering of the traveler, who was beaten and abandoned, evoked a caring, loving response from the Good Samaritan. That exchange of love would not have occurred if the traveler had not suffered, and if the Good Samaritan had not recognized that suffering and stopped to help. What Pope John Paul is telling us is this: "Suffering is present in the world in order to release love, in order to give birth to works of love towards neighbour, in order to transform the whole of human civilization into a 'civilization of love.'"[26] The Good Samaritan can be considered a figure of Christ, the inn to which He brought the traveler a figure of the Church, and the innkeeper the priest. Yes, it is difficult when patients come to me with their suffering, but if I can connect with them in a loving way and help them deal with their suffering, then I too help release love into the world.

My home parish is St. Paul's in Harvard Square. The parish serves the Harvard community and has a boys' choir school and a men's schola. I enjoy the wonderful music there, but I also love meeting the parishioners and trying to influence people with good where I can.

For years part of my role in the parish was just to get my mother to Mass. She died three years ago, at the age of nearly 100. As long as her health permitted, she was a daily communicant. We went to Mass together every Sunday, with her in her wheelchair, until just a few weeks before she died. After Mass we'd always attend the coffee hour, as I still do now. She had many friends there. Young people would come to talk with her, help with her wheelchair and with transfers in and out of the car.

Her death was written up in the Boston Globe, because she had been well-known in Boston as a pioneering female doctor. Our pastor couldn't celebrate the funeral because of a scheduling conflict, so I asked our former pastor, Bishop John Boles. He had also been on the board of our hospice. He had called me when Mother was admitted to hospice and asked me to let him know if he could do anything to help. He graciously accepted my invitation to celebrate her funeral Mass. I was amazed that morning to see seven other priests on the altar concelebrating with him.

Until she died, I didn't realize how much the care of my mother impressed the people in my parish. Her witness in attending Mass despite her infirmity, and my witness in caring for her to the end, seemed to be very important to many, many people. The

---

26. Pope John Paul II, encyclical. *On the Meaning of Human Suffering* (*Salvifici Dolores*); 30: 1984.

funeral director who arranged the services suggested that, since Mother had been so old and my sister lived so far away, we wouldn't need more than 50 holy cards for the funeral. "How about 300?" I replied. So we ordered 300, and every single one of them was taken.

I'm no longer active in hospice, but when my mother was ill, I called Good Samaritan, which I helped found, and the staff helped me care for my mother during her last weeks. Hospice's support and medications were wonderful and for me, it was like coming full circle. A hospice nurse was with us at the house on my mother's last night. She was restless and I knew from experience that if we prayed the rosary she would settle down. As she could no longer respond to the prayers, I asked the nurse if she would like to pray the rosary with me. She said that although she was not Catholic she had learned the rosary in Catholic school in Rwanda. We prayed it together and then I prayed the prayers for the dying, which the priest had left for us earlier that day after he gave Mother the Sacrament of the Sick. The nurse found them so beautiful that she asked for a copy of the prayers to share with other families. As we prayed, Mother became very peaceful. After a short time her breathing became slower and shallower. We called my sister who had been resting in the next room. My sister and I held her hands and told her that we hoped to join her and Dad in heaven one day. Without any struggle or discomfort, our Mother died peacefully.

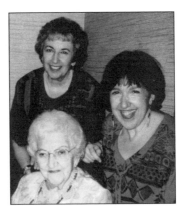

90th Birthday Celebration: June 10, 1996
Dr. E. Joanne Angelo, Carolyn Angelo (standing)
Eda Polcari Angelo (seated)

— Ad Majorem Dei Gloriam —

6

Dr. Allan Ramey

ONE STEP
IN HEAVEN

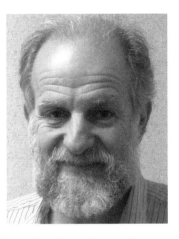

I was born in Lawrence, Massachusetts; my parents were Lebanese. I was raised in the Maronite Catholic Church, one of the Eastern Rite Catholic Churches that are faithful to the Pope but still retain a very eastern form of liturgy and worship. We date back to the Church's first mission in Antioch. Our first bishop was Peter—he came to Antioch before he went to Rome.

The Maronite Church was named after St. Maron, a fourth-century monk whose teachings paralleled those of St. Anthony of Egypt, the Desert Father. Maron's monastic order re-established the Christian faith throughout the region of Lebanon north of Palestine. The order's work was similar to what St. Benedict did in re-establishing Western civilization and Christianity after the barbarian invasions in Europe. The Maronite Church retains that sense of the monastic.

I first really understood something about my faith when I was serving as an altar boy, in about second grade. Most of our Masses were in Aramaic, the ancient language of Our Lord. I began to get a sense of faith listening to the women of the choir as they sang, their voices wailing, especially for the Stations of the Cross during Lent. Even though the words were beyond my understanding, I experienced a sense of awe and great reverence for God.

I began to understand little pieces of the language, and realized that the Aramaic word, ירא, "yirah," is always attached to the name of God, Yahweh. Yirah means fear, but not the fear that we think about when we're in dread or startled. It refers to fear in the sense of deep respect, awe, reverence and wonder.[27]

---

27. For more see: Michael Anthony (a.k.a. Brother Anthony Opisso), *The Book of Understanding*. Benyamin Publishers, 1994.

As I grew older, I became more exposed to the Latin Rite and came to love the Latin Mass too. When, as a third grader, I heard the news that the Latin Mass would no longer be prayed, I thought that someone in Rome had gone crazy. I went home that day and took my Latin Missal, which was a gift from my aunt Vivian, and hid it. I was afraid that people might forget; that we might lose the Mass! I still love the Latin Mass. In it, I find all the teachings of the Church. Though not thoroughly absent from the New Order of the Mass, these teachings aren't so clearly and unambiguously taught there. In the Latin Mass there is a sense of reverence and deep understanding or תבונה, "tebunah."

I was already going to daily Mass when I started undergraduate work at Harvard. I had an interest in the sciences, but my plan of study was not initially geared toward becoming a physician. By the midpoint of my college years, I decided that medicine would be a good option for me, and I began to actively pursue it. But living a year in Harvard Yard does a lot to a person. I had to physically leave my family and my church and was immersed in a culture of depravity. In the 1970s, Harvard was all about deconstructing everything that had been built up before, about breaking down every shred of decency and tradition, and demonstrating to students that their cultural background was nothing but foolishness. For me, it was a hell on earth.

In my first year there, I witnessed young men gang-raping a young woman who was drunk. I witnessed athletes and other talented young people drinking themselves into oblivion. There was so much unsupervised debauchery that when I was a sophomore, I petitioned to be allowed to live off campus. Permission was granted, despite the hard and fast rule that underclassmen must live on campus. I think the administration was afraid of what I wrote in my petition, of the potential for public scandal.

So in a way I stayed at Harvard, but I didn't stay. I continued my coursework but lived for my remaining years in a charismatic prayer community in Brighton, with a group of men from different walks of life. We had prayer together every morning and attended Mass daily on the Boston College campus. After dinner we'd convene again for night prayer. We had a brotherhood, a short-term agreement to live in this monastic way, which allowed me to stay focused on my faith as I attended school. But at the same time this was an eternal covenant, for I loved these men and over the years have remained connected with them by letter and by prayer.

My wife, Marita, and I met while I was living in Brighton; we dated for a couple of years before we were married.

I recognized early on at Harvard that there was no teacher there who had the capability to teach the most important thing in all of life: the Truth. I was working part-time as a janitor and one day after I finished washing the floors, I sat in my closet on an upturned bucket, a bare light bulb above me, and my Bible in my hands. I said, "Lord, I don't understand this. Holy Spirit, be my teacher. There's no one here to teach me Your Word."

That very day, the Holy Spirit honored that prayer. The meaning of the Scripture verses I had read that morning was revealed to me through the circumstantial events of the day. Things began to connect, and my life became a day-by-day walk with God. I kept reading Scripture, asking God to direct my reading, and often found that what I was directed to read was taught and expanded on at that day's Mass. As a result of His direction, questions would come up that would be answered as I went along. I asked the Holy Spirit to be my teacher, and I've been enrolled as His student ever since.

I kept reading and learning through my years in medical school at the University of Massachusetts. I made the decision not to pursue the surgery track because by then my wife, Marita, and I had a growing family, and surgery didn't seem like a plausible option for me. So, instead, I decided to become an internist, caring for adults. During my training in internal medicine, I became interested in rheumatologic illnesses. Eventually I limited my practice to rheumatology so that I could work a 40-hour week, without a lot of night call, and could respond to the needs of my family.

My work as a physician is a continuous conversation about healing that goes on in 15-minute vignettes throughout the day in my busy practice. The Lord sends me individuals who have medical needs but who also need to converse about faith or family, hope or despair. My job is to pray for God to give me שׂכל, "sakal"— a Hebrew word for the understanding of what to do next. That is what Joshua prayed for at the walls of Jericho and that is what I pray for when a patient comes to me.

If a patient comes in with a swollen knee, during those 15 minutes as I drain the joint and inject some medication, we talk. The knee just led them into the conversation. A person could do the same thing as a bartender, barber, or lawyer—you name it. The vocations, as I see them, provide us with a vehicle through which we can engage in battle and help others gain faith, hope and forgiveness.

I think it's foolishness for Catholics in any profession to think that they are going to be able to put their faith in a box and not exercise it in their daily life. If you understand that God reigns and that His word is Truth, how can you not bring that word into your arena? I don't care if you go to a rock 'n' roll party; you'd better bring your Christian faith with you. And if you have a conversation in the midst of that noise, it had better be a Christian one that brings people to a better place. Faith should not be isolated. It should be brought into public places where sinners live and work and play. You should be bringing faith with you, just as Jesus did. That's what was done for us. We need only to extend that courtesy.

Sometimes when I identify myself as a Catholic, a patient says, "Why do you go to *that* church? I was Catholic once, but they're a bunch of hypocrites." "Well," I say, "I'm a hypocrite too. We're all sinners. The Church is made up of sinners. If you go into a bar, there are hypocrites there also." This puts things into perspective for them.

But in our culture today, we're constantly asked to compromise our faith. The state of Massachusetts doesn't want me to talk about my faith in the context of my medical practice. In medical school, I got the message that this was considered unprofessional. In reality the culture is trying to indoctrinate us with what amounts to a secular, atheistic ideology. But that's a religion as well. And secularists frequently attempt to oppress others with their very restrictive world-view.

It's commonly held that applying Catholic principles in medicine means that you're not applying scientific principles. That's not the case at all. It's not a question of being antiscientific in order to be holy and Catholic. Science is perfected in understanding the revelation of God that is found in humanity. Science outside this context of holy covenant is lost. In our current state of moral breakdown, financial concerns override all others. No one is standing as a moral governor. God has revealed to us that some actions are immoral. God teaches us. He's trying all He can to teach us a moral code, through every vehicle possible, in any way we will listen. And the fruit of obedience is a covenant relationship, a bond forever between the human and the Divine.

The Catholic Church has been the propagator of some of the finest scientific principles through the ages. Catholic scientists and physicians have made many discoveries that are important in my own work as a physician, including Pasteur and his work in bacteriology, Laennec who invented the stethoscope, and Mendel who did pioneering work in genetics. The concept of deductive reasoning and the research techniques of double-blinded controlled trials and prospective trials all came out of the Catholic love for honesty and truth. Those who love the truth recognize that when we do research we are subject to bias, so research needs to be blinded. It's faith that insists that science remains true, that we don't go by personal bias or hearsay, because the outcomes are too important. People's lives are at stake.

The Old Testament book of Sirach (Ecclesiasticus) gives this advice: "Obey the physician, because he prays daily and receives counsel from God."[28] The Scripture places physicians in a position of authority and this is not based on the fact that they are educated and have medical degrees, but on the fact that they pray. So my day begins in prayer at a brief New Order Mass at 6:30 a.m. at St. Cecilia's Church in Leominster. I try my best to bring to it that sensibility from the Latin Mass, so that I don't forget the awe, the role of the priest, the fact that God wants us to be one with Him, the fact that Christ is present in the Eucharist. And then I receive Communion.

I think of Our Lady and I try to emulate her. She is the perfect mother, the perfect spouse, and the perfect daughter to God in the Trinitarian relationship. So like her, I need to be a spouse of God—like a bride I give my desires and my will to Him. I say, "All for You, Lord. Show me what's next." I also need to be a son of God, to hear His word, to listen very carefully and make it part of me. Finally, I need to be a mother of God. I do it by bringing Christ into the world, into these circumstances, into this need, every day.

So after Mass, when I come back to get my children ready for school or go to my office for my patients, I need to try to bring Christ to them, to bring Him into the world around me. That's my job as a warrior in the battle God calls us to fight against evil. That's the basis of my life at work and with my family.

People bring me their needs, not just their arthritis. They bring their tears about their families, their estrangements from one another, their despair, their sins, their need for virtue. So I engage them in prayer and conversation.

---

28. Sir 38:12-14

The patients seem to respond to this. The younger ones will say it like this: "I don't know why, but whenever I come here I feel better." They don't know exactly what's happening, but they know there's something good here and they return for more. The older patients know exactly what's going on. They're in a life of prayer also, praying daily Mass. They're part of the battle. So they come and we have an intellectual conversation. It helps sort things out and I learn from them as well.

Once in a while I send someone out with a particular word, usually from Scripture. If the patient has a problem that won't go away, for instance, I might ask them to think about Naaman from the Old Testament, who had leprosy.[29] When he sought healing, God asked a very small thing of Naaman. Through Elijah the prophet, God told Naaman to go to the Jordan River and bathe in it seven times, and he'd be clean.

Naaman was insulted. His response was, "Are not the rivers of Damascus, the Abana and the Pharpar, better than all the waters of Israel?" He was about to return to Syria when his slave girl, who loved him, pointed out, "If the prophet had told you to do something extraordinary, would you not have done it? All the more now, since he said to you, 'Wash and be clean,' should you do as he said." And I'm sure she begged him tearfully. So out of love for her, he swallowed his pride and followed the prophet's instructions, and he was healed of his leprosy.

So sometimes healing requires a simple thing that God can work with. I may tell a patient to go and say a prayer before the Eucharist at St. John Church down the street, because the Eucharist is exposed there for adoration. So the person might go and sit there before the Eucharist even if she's never done that before. She might not even be Catholic. But she'll say, "Okay, God, if You're here, will You please let me know. What can You show me?" And all manner of things happen.

I don't think I've met a patient who doesn't have a lesson to offer me. Sometimes I'm most surprised at some of my young ones who have particular conditions they suffer with, such as juvenile rheumatoid arthritis. They're so capable of bringing lightheartedness to our sessions; I really enjoy them. And from my older patients, the most interesting thing I get is a historical perspective. I ask my patients in their 90s what they remember—they're like walking history lessons. They tell me stories of where they were and

---

29. 2 Kings 5:1-19

what they were doing during World War II, and it gives me more insight into them as persons, like opening a treasure chest.

When my wife, Marita, and I were first married our life was one of walking in faith together. We had our daughter Jessica after we'd been married a year and a half. From that point on our marriage was all about how to raise kids and apply Catholic principles. We began to realize very quickly that it's not always clear which way is the right way. Figuring that out wasn't easy, even though we were both Catholic, because the culture is so anti-Catholic. We differed on matters such as what is enough immersion into the culture and what is too much protection.

For example: is Disney all right? Walt Disney, Mr. Benign for kids. If Disney is on the label, it's okay for kids—that's what I was raised to accept. But Disney was a naturalist and his movies teach that there's power in nature, for good and for evil. According to the Disney philosophy, what power serves your own purpose is good, and what thwarts your purpose is evil.

Marita and I would have conversations about this. She thought a lot with her heart, and she saw Disney as just enjoyment for the children, and sometimes that's the way we went. That's okay. God gives us a lot of leeway. We have to be patient with ourselves, as He is with us. I suppose ultimately the truth wins out.

Even in high school, our daughter Jessica had a strong faith. She went to a Catholic school and once she told me about a speaker who came to their assembly, a very unfortunate man who was a homosexual and had contracted AIDS. He'd been invited there to give a talk on how to have "safe sex" through mutual masturbation. Basically, he was teaching scandal. When Jessica told us about it, Marita and I went down there to hear his second presentation for ourselves. The high school faculty was saying that what the speaker had to say was difficult, but we needed to hear it. They tried to silence any comments from the audience and intimidate anybody who tried to leave.

One of the mothers in the audience put up her hand and asked the speaker a very interesting question: "Have you ever known someone with AIDS who was cured by prayer?" He said that he had; he'd noticed that sometimes people's health did improve when they prayed. I wondered how I could take the next step. The mother had asked a very good question and she got an intriguing and thoughtful answer from him. So I put up my hand and asked, "Would you be interested in us praying for you, that you would be healed?" Immediately, the teachers intervened, saying it was time for sports practice. But I persisted. "Would you like us to pray for you?" The speaker said, "Yes, I would."

"The man asked for prayers," I told the teachers. "So can we do this?" I guess I was shaming them. So I went onto the stage with my wife and the lady who asked the first question. I called out to the school counselor and the teaching nuns and said, "How about you joining us too?" And there we stood all around the man with our hands on his head. I prayed that God would help him, that He would give him peace and teach him the truth. I made it a point to also pray that he might be a light in the darkness and bring the truth to people and not personal opinion or prejudice against the Church.

Jessica's high school friends were all confused. Later they said to her, "I thought your father was against this guy. But he was helping him!" I asked her, "What did you say to your friends about that?"

She told me she had answered, "That's Catholicism, I guess." That was the best answer she could have given to those kids who didn't really understand what the Faith is. This was an issue of faith and morals, and someone had to make a statement.

I heard that the speaker never gave another talk, and died shortly thereafter. Hopefully he died in peace. Like most zealots, he thought he was doing a good thing. But when you fall away from the real teaching of the Church, you're doing great harm. Perhaps he knows that now.

Marita and I had eight children. Our sixth child, Sarah, we adopted as an infant from Lebanon. If you lined up all of my children and I asked you which one was adopted, you'd never pick her. I like to tell Sarah that she and I are the only pureblooded Lebanese in the family, that the other children are half Irish. I take the fact of our similar looks as a sign of our God-inspired destiny together. In reality, there are no pureblooded Lebanese. Much like Americans, we are a melting pot of cultures, a mixture of Arab, Phoenician, Turk, Jew, and Greek.

Sarah's adoption came about through direction and prayer to St. Joseph, the patron of families. God wanted this little girl here. It was very directed; I even knew her name. Marita would ask me, "Can we go on vacation to Disneyland?" Disneyland, of all places! "Well," I'd answer, "if we really have to go to Disneyland, I don't want to go yet. I want to wait until Sarah comes so we can take her too." She'd say, "Who's Sarah?" and I'd answer, "You know, our next kid." She'd tell me, "Be quiet. She is *not* going to be called Sarah." I guess in a way I was tormenting her with this. As a child, Marita knew a little girl named Sarah who used to fight with her all the time, so she didn't want that name. And I would frustrate her so much with my insistence.

Marita and I always felt the need to give back to society. She wanted to be sure that our efforts were going to do some real good, that we weren't just sending money to a charity with big administrative expenses. So she suggested, "Why don't we do something we can see right here?" We finally agreed that adoption would be a good way to see the effects of our work. So we pursued the process and found a Melkite nun, Mother Antonia, who ran an orphanage in Lebanon. She came and interviewed us.

Eventually we got a phone call in our bedroom in the middle of the night. Mother Antonia said they had a two-day-old baby for us. I asked her, "What's the baby's name?" She answered, "How do you like the name Christine?"

I said, "Hold on a second." I told Marita, "Mother Antonia wants to know if you like Christine for a name." "Yeah," she said. "I like that name." So I said, "Marita likes that name, that's fine." I kind of wondered internally about it, but I didn't say anything.

Getting the baby out of Lebanon was a challenge. We couldn't even get *into* Lebanon. This was during the height of the hostage crisis in Lebanon in which Terry Waite and others were being held by Islamic terrorists. There was a ban on travel and no U.S. citizens were being allowed into Lebanon. We were told that if we got in by some illegal means, we wouldn't be allowed out of the country and if the baby was found with us, she would be sent back to the orphanage. We didn't understand how we were going to get her out. After four months of prayer and trial, finally God figured out a way for her to be released to Cyprus. We made all the arrangements, went to Cyprus, but when we went to pick up the baby, again we failed and had to return to the United States. We tried again only Marita went alone, and this time she succeeded.

So after so much frustration and failed efforts, finally Marita was sitting in a hotel in Nicosia, rocking the baby. I can see it in my mind now, even though I wasn't there. She was cooing, "Oh Christine, I love you," and the lady who had brought her the baby said, "It's strange to hear you calling her Christine. We haven't been calling her by that name." Marita asked, "What have you been calling her?"

"Well," the woman admitted, "she was given another name when she was born. But Mother Antonia asked your husband about naming her Christine because she thought it sounded more American. We've been calling her Sarah."

Marita nearly dropped the baby! Later, when Mother Antonia arrived, Marita asked, "Have you been talking to Allan?" She said no, and told her to tell me that this was the baby God had chosen for us. Later I told Marita I was okay with the name Christine.

About a month later, I bumped into a priest who had prayed for Marita and me on our first trip out to Cyprus—very specific prayers, about the Angel Raphael guiding our travels and helping us bring back the one who was promised. I told him we had the baby and her name was Christine. He said to me, "Her name is Sarah!"

I was a little startled, but to tell you the truth, nothing surprises me in faith any longer. "Don't you know who Sarah is?" he asked.

I said, "Sure. She's Abraham's wife in the Old Testament."

He said, "Not that Sarah—the Sarah from the book of Tobias, the one whom Tobias saved and brought back to his family. Have Marita come to me."

When I told Marita "Father Carroll wants to see you," and explained why, she admitted that the visit would be unnecessary. "Never mind. We'll change her name back to Sarah."

Boy, talk about a pain in the neck. We had to fill out a lot of paperwork just to change her name! You don't need faith when things like that happen around you constantly. You do, however, need prayer. Every day you need prayer.

People often ask why we adopted when we already had children of our own. Most couples adopt a child because of infertility. I've realized that some people can't have children because God has a specific child for them. Infertile couples somehow get referred to my practice after they've tried all the assisted reproduction techniques at all the local hospitals and specialty centers. They tell me, "Somebody said you have a way of helping us." I tell them, "Well, I don't have a way. But maybe God needs a family for a particular child, someone for whom you'd make really good parents, someone you could adopt. Why don't you pursue that first? Pray and see if that could be true. Go to an agency and start the process. See what happens." So many times, they adopt a child and a year or two later they get pregnant.

So including Sarah, we had eight children. Our oldest daughter Jessica was a very, very pretty girl, petite and attractive. She had young men all around her from an early age. They were infatuated with her, and she would often bring them with us to church. They'd follow her anywhere, even to church. She told me, "Dad, that's my job."

I would challenge her a lot on this. "Don't flaunt your beauty," I told her. "Maybe this 'ministry' of yours isn't the right ministry for you. A young woman having a ministry to young men? That would be like me going into the Combat Zone in Boston, to minister to the prostitutes and strippers. That would be a job for your grandma, not for me."

She would laugh at that, because her grandma was a powerful Catholic lady who went out into the cold at age 80 to march and got arrested at pro-life demonstrations. But Jessica didn't change her mind. She said, "I understand what you're saying, but this is what I need to do because it works." I think she had a real awareness of what God wanted, how to use that gift of physical beauty that so many other women would see as a curse.

She continued to do that until she died tragically in a motor vehicle accident when she was only 19. And at her wake, don't you know, all those young men, one after another, came to pay their respects.

Jessica died on her way back home from college at Franciscan University of Steubenville. Stephen, her boyfriend of a year, was driving. This was in the pre-airbag era. She probably didn't have a seat belt on either. She rarely used her seatbelt. I rarely did either.

They were making a detour to avoid some construction in Scranton, Pennsylvania. Stephen was making a left turn from that middle turning lane that the highways down there have, and he saw another car coming the other direction, also making a left turn. So he figured it was safe for him to turn too. Stephen didn't see another car coming at about 60 miles per hour. The driver had had a couple of beers with his lunch; he was just below the established legal limit. He plowed into the side of their vehicle. Jessica died instantly—she had a broken neck—her head and shoulders were driven into the windshield.

Stephen survived, thanks be to God. He probably had stronger bones than Jessica. He wound up in the hospital for quite a while, and then he came and stayed with us for a week. He had little recollection of the accident and at one point he mustered up the courage to ask whose fault it was. I simply explained the details to him as well as I could. And I told Stephen that we will see wisdom one day in even the permissive will of God, not only in His providential will.

Jessica's boyfriend, Stephen, still visits us periodically. Some years ago he got married, and he told us about it almost apologetically. I said, "Don't be worried. You had no vow with Jessica. She's blessing you from heaven."

When he and his wife had their first child, he wanted to name the baby Jessica, but his wife wouldn't allow it. Instead, she picked the name Grace. I told the young man, "I want you to understand that 'grace' is the meaning of the name Jessica in Hebrew. So you can be consoled. Your wife doesn't have to worry. She's the one who picked the name." He was really grateful for that.

We established a foundation in Jessica's honor using the life insurance settlement we received, and we use the funds for mission trips to the Dominican Republic and Haiti.[30] It was more or less to put it back in the devil's face—to say, "Well, you took this life, but some of its purpose will still be fulfilled." Jessica herself had wanted to go do mission work in the Caribbean. She had a friend from Jamaica who told her of the problems with poverty down there and the need for help. Jessica had a heart for the people of the Islands. She collected surplus medicines from our office and packed them up for shipment to the Caribbean.

Jessica's friends picked up on the mission work too. They knew she would have had a profound effect on these poor children so now they are going in her place. The kids who want to come with us on these trips first have to pray about it. I ask them about their prayer life and encourage them to expand on it: If they already pray at night, I suggest that they add a daily rosary; if they go to Sunday Mass, I encourage them to try to go daily. I want them to see what God is telling them, to see if they're being called to mission work. One out of every three young persons who asks me about the work decides to go and by that time, they are very grounded in prayer.

Prayer is really the missing ingredient in so much work for social justice. We have to be listening to the General to see what should be done; otherwise our work is redundant or counterpro-

---

30. Jessica Marie Ramey Catholic Charitable Foundation

ductive. That which we judge as "good," is not necessarily God's judgment. But He is the one doing real good through us. Sometimes when we look back, we are graced to see that what we did was really necessary and also that other people were hearing the Word and doing complementary things. We can see that there's a coordinated effort. We can see that God really is in charge.

People ask me how we can do anything when we go down to the mission for just a week at a time and have so little money. Well, I respond, we've managed to accomplish a great many things. In just four days we built a church, a school, and a clinic in Haiti outside Pignon, thanks to the relationship I've built up with a priest there and a concept God put in the priest's mind. Now 4,000 people in the village have a school and a church.

In one of the barrios of Santo Domingo, we completed a church for the neighborhood. We were able to provide housing for 56 families in Constanza. We'd gone there to bring medicines, and we found young girls asking for antibiotics for infections. Our interpreter discovered that these girls had vaginal infections. The community was so dysfunctional that men from the village were systematically raping the young girls. Their mothers had no clue about this; there was no policing.

We made some inquiries with the local priest about how we could get these girls and their families out of that environment. He told us they had tried to raise money to build houses for the villagers, but they'd only raised enough to build two houses.

"How much is a house?" I asked him. He told me that with $700 in US funds they could construct a concrete house with two rooms and a porch, a strong, hurricane-proof metal roof, all painted, very pretty, a dignified place to live. The church had the land to build on, he said.

I said, "Okay. If I can find you the money, can you build these houses and select the families who need them?" He said yes. This was all negotiated in one week.

I came back and wrote letters to 40 or 50 friends and got 20 letters in return. In each of those 20 letters was a check for $700 to cover the cost of one house. I sent the money to Constanza, and then more money began trickling in. With the money donated we were able to build new houses as well as repair some existing homes to make them livable. We sent pictures of the families to our donors, so they could see whom they helped as a result of their generosity. So now 56 families have safe places to live. They have employment; they're working to support themselves. Some of them have even prospered enough to add on to their houses.

I can't get my head around how any of that happened. That's God's work. God just put us in a place and showed us the problem. He already knew the solution.

Six years after Jessica's accident, my wife Marita died. That was September 8, 2001, the Nativity of the Blessed Virgin Mary, three days before the Twin Towers went down. We had been married 26 years. That was a frightening week for the whole country, wasn't it? She'd had a checkup shortly before, and everything seemed fine. There was nothing anybody could have done— it was sudden and unexpected. I think it was finally determined that she had a dissection of the aorta. We did CPR. We did everything we could. We brought her heart back to a normal rhythm seven times, and seven times she went back down. I told the children later that Mom was struggling against God's will, begging Him to let her stay. She did that once for each child that was here.

But she had one child in heaven too, and that was good. I know Jessica received her.

Our youngest child, Simeon, was just a baby when his mom passed away. He received a holy vision of his mother in glory. It was an answer to a prayer. We had asked God to help us explain to a two-year-old that his mother wasn't coming back. I had no clue what to do for him. He just cried and cried his heart out every morning because I came to him instead of his mother. The crying started the first morning after Marita's death, when I went to get him from his crib. When Mom didn't come, he became angry and looked at me as if it was my fault, and he cried and cried in anger. This went on every morning for a week.

On the seventh day of this, I brought him downstairs and rocked him and rocked him. It was 5:00 a.m. My head drooped back; I didn't know what to do to make him better. I didn't know what to do at all. Suddenly, he startled me by breaking into laughter—crazy laughter. Patrick, his brother, was lying on the couch near us—he'd been too anxious to sleep in his own room— and he'd pulled his pillow over his head because he didn't want to hear Simeon cry. Now, when Patrick heard the laughter, he put the pillow down and asked me, "Is he dreaming?" I didn't know. I thought maybe he was having a seizure. I didn't really know what was going on, why he was laughing so much.

Then I looked more closely at his little face. His eyes were transfixed on something, which seemed to be located in mid air in the middle of the room. Neither Patrick nor I saw anything, but Simeon's eyes were wide. Every couple of seconds, his pupils enlarged and he giggled out loud. Then he'd stop, look some more in anticipation, then giggle again as his eyes got wider. It was just like what he used to do when his mom played peek-a-boo with him. Now he was seeing his mom in a glorified state. After a few minutes it was over. Simeon looked at me, and asked for something to eat.

It was the most unbelievable thing I ever saw in my life. Patrick said to me, "Dad, if people see something like this, how could they believe that there is no God?" I told Patrick, "I'm just so happy that you're here, because no one would believe me. It takes two to bear witness to the truth."

That day was September 15th, the feast of Our Lady of Sorrows, and that vision was what God gave Simeon to help him through his pain. The next morning he didn't cry. He never cried again, looking for Mom.

The Blessed Mother came to Simeon in the vision with Marita that day too. I know this because afterwards he would look at a picture of Mary and say, "Ma!" I would say, "No, that's not your mom. Here's a picture of your mom." And he'd say "Yeah, Ma," and he would point to it and then he'd point back to the picture of Mary and say, "Ma." He understood that they were both his mom; that Mary was going to be his Mother through his life, and his mother Marita was going to be with him too. That's a true story.

Now we walk every day with one step on earth and one step in heaven. We have family both here and there. But we're unified, just like the Church. We have the Church Militant on earth and the Church Triumphant in glory in heaven, and it's the same Church. We team up together, and we both pray for the Church in purgatory, which is suffering.

People ask me if I'm angry with God. I think anger with God presupposes that we have a better plan than His. I don't. I feel that this is a strange question from a perspective of faith. I am in pain at the loss, but anger has no place in that pain. If anger were a part of it I would pray for the virtue of fortitude to overcome the deadly disposition. This is what happens—we suffer, we die, we go to heaven. The timing? That's God's will, not mine.

I suppose if I wasn't walking in the faith or receiving the Sacraments, I'd be a very different man. I know I'd be feeling sorry for myself, saying things like, "What kind of God would tear the heart out of a family? A family needs its mother!"…all that kind of nonsense. That comes from self-pity, from a place that's human "wisdom." Such thoughts have nothing to do with the reality of things.

Instead, for me reality was just persisting in the Faith. The receiving of the Blessed Sacrament daily provided me with power to persevere through the mourning period and the reframing of our lives together. Instead of being a self-absorbed man, through the Sacraments, I was perhaps overwhelmed, but not angry. The Sacraments gave me fortitude. Every day I'd go to Mass early and come back just in time to get the kids ready for school and on their way. We had some friends who helped and picked them up, because the children were going in four different directions to different schools. I went to work, completed my duties and then returned home in time to help them with homework, make supper, give them their baths, and get them all to bed.

And then at about midnight I'd be folding clothes. That's what I usually did at the end of the day. At that point, everything in the house was quiet, and I'd be thinking about the children as I folded their clothes. Mothers must do this too. I'd fold Jesse's shirt or Rachel's dress, and I'd pray for each. And I'd feel this kind of presence. Marita was with me expressing her profound gratitude for taking such good care of her children.

It was the most peculiar thing. I never considered that I deserved gratitude from her for taking care of our own children. But that's exactly what I was feeling. I could feel her saying, "Thank you for taking good care of them." So I knew that, even then, I wasn't abandoned, that she was there and God was there.

I've shared about this with my elderly patients who have lost someone they love, and they understand, they know. My patients tell me one story after another like this. I guess something about the doctor-patient interaction gives them a vehicle to tell me their stories.

One woman who lost her husband told me she was so put off by all the tubes in him during his last illness in the hospital that she was afraid to disturb anything. "My only regret," she told me, "was that I didn't kiss him goodbye."

"So one night after he died," she continued, "I woke from sleep and felt the bed go down, as if he was getting in. I turned a little and felt something press my lips. I opened my eyes and nobody was there."

I hear so many stories like that from people who are Catholics in good faith, who love God. They just need that little bit of help so they can persevere, so they can perceive that the faith they've put in the Word of God is not in vain. They need to have hope in what will come to pass—true hope. This was the hope that we see in the Blessed Virgin Mary: "And blessed are you who believed that what was spoken to you by the Lord would be fulfilled."[31]

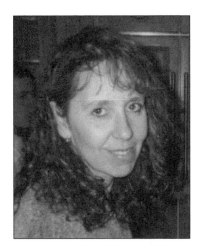

Marita Ramey

— Ad Majorem Dei Gloriam —

---

31. Luke 1:45

7

Dr. Harvey Clermont

THE SURGEON'S SILVER LINING

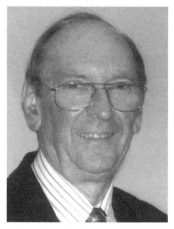

I was born into the Catholic Church and raised in the predominantly Catholic town of Adams, Massachusetts, up in the Berkshires. My mother was Polish and my father French, and each nationality had its own Catholic Church and school in the town. We went to the French Church, and in those days, everything at Mass was either in Latin or French. My father and mother ran a grocery store, but she was actually the mainstay of the business because he was so busy with community work. When we were growing up, my three younger sisters and I helped out a lot at the grocery.

Adams was a blue-collar mill town and its economy was dependent on the textile mills. It was not unusual in those days for children—and they really were children—to go to work in the mills when they reached the age of 16. If they were fortunate and could get a little more schooling, they might get a better job on the assembly line at Sprague Electric in North Adams or at General Electric in Pittsfield. Most of the children at that time didn't leave town, unless they went into the military. Since the United States had conscription at the time, all the boys had to sign up when they turned 18. In a way, we didn't have a lot of choices but that was the way it was.

If you were Catholic, you went to church and that too, was the way it was. Apart from Mass, there were very few activities at church—nothing like what exists now. There was no parish council so the priests basically ran the parishes. There wasn't a lot of lay involvement either. In general, the people who got involved in the parish were women; they ran the fundraisers, the bake sales, and such things.

From kindergarten through eighth grade, I attended a parochial school run by the Sisters of Our Lady of Seven Dolors, a French Canadian order. They were strict disciplinarians as most teachers were in those days. But that was beneficial, so I don't look back at that as a bad time. I think the organizational skills and the faith they taught were, in retrospect, very good for us. It made us strong and molded our lives in positive ways.

In first grade, I became an altar boy. I enjoyed doing that—it got me out of school! We got called periodically to do weddings or funerals in the middle of the school day and since I was a good student, the teachers didn't mind letting me out. So every now and then off I went on these little hiatuses. We also had frequent processions on feast days—they were a big thing. Perhaps the biggest each year was on May 1, in honor of the Virgin Mary. Students from the two Catholic schools, one Polish and the other French, marched in a parade through the center of town carrying the blue and white banners.

I was one of four of my grade school classmates who attended St. Joseph High School. The others attended public school. Since St. Joseph was in North Adams, I either had to thumb rides or pedal a bike five miles to school. The nuns who taught us were extremely well educated, each having the equivalent of a master's or doctoral degree. They provided us an education in the Jesuit tradition, which is strongly rooted in the classics and philosophy. I took four years of Latin and two years of Greek, which led to my interest in languages. Today I speak Spanish, which was partly stimulated by my early language education.

Our coursework was also very strong in English. I participated in competitions with other Catholic schools in spelling bees and in contests regarding word root derivatives. The only areas in which St. Joseph was weak were science and math. Of course, I didn't find that out until I went to college and had to catch up, but in language, literature, and the humanities, I was far ahead.

After St. Joseph, I attended the College of the Holy Cross in Worcester, Massachusetts, also a Jesuit school. At that time, only men were admitted but it has since become co-educational. Again, they were a little weak in science but *par excellence* in the classics. We studied Thomas Aquinas in philosophy and had to take theology courses as well. The Jesuits prepared us for all professions, from medicine to business to law. A Jesuit education taught you to think differently from the approach used at Ivy League schools. The

Ivies allowed students to think on their own, without studying the great minds of the past and how their thought processes evolved. In contrast, the Jesuit approach was to study those past thinkers first, then to allow us to choose what we thought were the important elements in their thought processes.

In my ethics class, we learned syllogisms. Frequently I would argue, "A is correct but B doesn't seem to be correct, so I can't come to C." That would start a fight. I was always kind of independent in thought, and I rebelled at some of the organized thinking that they were banging into us. I wanted to break out of that pattern, but because of its natural logic, I found myself falling back on classical ways of thinking when I was in the secular world.

At Holy Cross I majored in biology but like many other students at that stage, I wasn't sure what I wanted to do after I graduated. I think it's good to be open-minded and to experience lots of different options, rather than narrowing your studies too early in life. I also experienced some personal tragedy while I was at Holy Cross when my father died the summer after my freshman year. Grieving, I wondered whether I should go back home, especially since I was the oldest in the family. But by September, I was at Holy Cross again.

At this point in my life, a lecture by Dr. Tom Dooley, a Catholic Navy lieutenant and physician, had a profound influence on me. In the 1950s he had been stationed on a Navy destroyer in Laos and got involved off the ship treating some of the local children and educating the Laotian physicians who had little exposure to modern medicine. When his tour of duty was over, he wanted to return to Laos, so he started a foundation called the Medical International Cooperation Organization (MEDICO), which worked to build hospitals in Southeast Asia.

Dooley's lecture fascinated me and stimulated me into thinking about a career in medicine. He lit a fire in me to go and do the kind of stuff he was doing. At the time he spoke at Holy Cross, Dooley was being treated for malignant melanoma. Ultimately the treatment was unsuccessful and he died a few years later. I was inspired to read some of Dooley's motivational books as well as the works of Albert Schweitzer. I was in awe of how much Schweitzer had given up, including a career as a virtuoso organist, to start a medical mission in the Congo. He had an extreme reverence for life—he cared for every living thing, whether plant, animal or insect. Most of us can't take it that far, but I understood his thought process nonetheless. The influence of Schweitzer and Dooley prompted me to go into medicine and sparked me to go beyond just seeing a patient, accepting a fee and moving on.

After Holy Cross I went to medical school at Harvard. I met a couple of surgeons there who had tremendous personalities. Because of the effortless way they did things, they had the respect of everyone. They also had a spirit of community service. Few people participated in voluntary missions at that time. Mostly it was the surgeons who went. Surgery lent itself well to short-term mission trips. You could go somewhere, perform surgery, train people in post-operative care, and do a lot of good for a lot of people in a short period of time. Some of the early mission surgeons were doing plastic surgeries, such as cleft palate repairs, which were life-saving for children whose deformities wouldn't allow them to eat.

Unlike my undergraduate education, at Harvard Medical School independent thought was highly valued. "Well, what do you think?" my professors would ask. My fellow students, who had come through a more liberal education process, often made arguments that weren't very substantial. But because I had studied the great thinkers of the past at Holy Cross, my arguments were more logic-based than emotion-based.

After Harvard I did my residency in general surgery at the University of Rochester. Our rotations included both psychiatry and medicine. I had the opportunity to do a lot of vascular surgery, since the chief at Rochester was a vascular surgeon. The hospital had a trauma center basically run by the surgical department, so I also got experience caring for patients with traumatic injuries.

By this time I was married with three children. I met Anne at a wedding, in which I was the best man, and as soon as I saw her, I knew I wanted to get together with her again. I don't think she felt the same way at first. At the time we met, she was a high school sophomore and I was a college sophomore. We got married about four years later and we moved to Boston. Our first child was born there and the next two arrived during my residency in Rochester.

It wasn't easy getting through residency with a family. In college I had worked three jobs: helping in a kitchen, delivering papers and delivering birthday cakes. As a result, my student loan debt at the end of college wasn't as bad as for many. During med school, to help pay the bills, I worked in a lab. Anne was very fortunate to get a job at the dean's office; she was allowed to bring the baby to work. He'd crawl around the office and the dean took a liking to him. I don't know for certain, but I suspect that might have been the reason I got a decent scholarship!

By the time I got to my surgical residency, I was working too many hours at the hospital to earn much money on the side. Back then the residents didn't have limited hours, as they do now. I was up every other night, and sometimes I'd go weeks before I got back home again. I was exposed to a lot and I learned a lot, but my schedule wasn't conducive to a good family life, that's for sure. All the other residents and their families were in the same boat, so most of the wives (there were very few female residents at that time) got together and socialized without their husbands. They supported each other and that got them through.

At the time, the draft for the Vietnam War was going on but I was fortunate enough to get a full deferment, which allowed me to finish my medical training. After my residency in Rochester, I went into the Navy for two years, figuring I'd end up in Southeast Asia—where else were they going to send a fully trained surgeon? But instead, I got orders to go to Alaska. One of the career Navy doctors up there decided he wanted to go to the war zone to further his career, and his move left a last-minute opening for a chief medical officer on a base in Alaska. It turned out to be two of the most memorable years of my life.

I was stationed in the town of Adak, Alaska, out on the Aleutian Islands. It was the westernmost town in the United States. Adak Naval Air Station was a very isolated base, but I really enjoyed being there, partly because I could feed my love of nature in that unique environment, a love nurtured by my years of growing up in the Berkshires. But it was a harsh environment and not a great place for bringing up a family so Anne and the children didn't enjoy it as much as I did.

I was head of the base hospital and enjoyed my interactions with the military personnel—I still keep in touch with some of them. I was impressed by their intense faith. The Catholics I met there tended to be very orthodox and strong in their beliefs. We had some lively philosophical and theological discussions. As I had done so often in college, I always took an opposing viewpoint, because I enjoyed egging them on. Sometimes I'd suggest a heretical idea, which would make them all nervous and upset. "How can you call yourself Catholic?" they would ask and I would reply, "Calm down. I just want you to think a little bit about what you believe. I'm trying to strengthen your belief, not tear it down." The give and take was fun because it reminded me of the dialogues in my ethics class at Holy Cross.

One of the best parts of my time in Alaska was the opportunity to participate in missions and deliver care to the native people who lived in remote villages. Many of the villages depended on what you might call shamans, who were basically elders with some knowledge of herbs or other life experience with health care. I was able to teach them some western medicine, and to take care of some of the villagers' medical problems as well. We were able to do a lot of good for people who were impoverished and had never been exposed to traditional Western medicine. My work there rekindled the flame of my original desire to become a doctor and I knew I wanted to do something like that again.

On the base, I regularly dealt with people with psychiatric problems. The isolation in Adak was intense and the enlisted men were there for a year at a time. Many were young without families and those who had families weren't able to bring them to Alaska. We had several suicides while I was there, which depressed the entire base. But I reached back into the training I'd had in psychiatry and I discovered that you could do a lot of good just by talking with people and re-directing their minds a little bit—probably as much good as I could do with a knife in surgery. I was grateful that my training had been broad enough to be helpful in that area.

Our base was located on one of the few sheltered deep-water harbors around. Many fishing vessels from different countries plied the fishing grounds offshore. They were allowed to fish outside a 20-mile limit but every now and then a boat would wander inside that limit and the Coast Guard would catch them, bring them into port, fine them, and then they'd head back out.

Once, a big Russian ship was pulled in. At that time, during the Cold War period, the Soviet health care system relied heavily on *feldshers*, who were the equivalent of nurse practitioners, for much of the primary care. Normally two or three *feldshers* traveled with the crew of these fishing vessels. This particular ship had two feldshers on staff. When one of them came down with acute abdominal pain, the other *feldsher* recognized that her colleague needed prompt attention. She put a call in to our base through an interpreter. Such calls were routinely monitored by the FBI and the KGB. Finally, the call came through to me and I was asked to see what I could do. Since boarding the Russian ship would have required special permission, I asked that the crew bring the patient to the base hospital.

She turned out to have an ectopic pregnancy. I operated on her that night and by the next day she was already feeling pretty decent. The other *feldsher* came to visit her in our hospital. She was smiling and everyone was happy. Through the interpreters, the *feldsher* invited me to go on board ship as a dinner guest of the captain. The KGB approved, so the next day my wife and I boarded the ship—along with our Secret Service agent, a KGB agent, and two interpreters.

We had been informed by one of the chiefs on our base that there were some things the Russians might like that they didn't have on board. "Bring 'em some Coca-Cola, some American magazines, and some fruit—they don't have any on board," he advised us. So we went to the commissary beforehand and picked up a case of Coke, some fruit, and some magazines. The Russian captain accepted our gifts graciously. Then he opened a big jug of vodka and filled our glasses. We only had a little, but one of the interpreters and the Secret Service agent were popping those drinks down one after another. By the time we finished our dinner and said goodbye, they were pretty well sloshed! Two days later, a judge in Anchorage was supposed to decide on the fine for violation of the off-shore limit by the Russian boat, but in the middle of the night, the captain just—pffft!—got the hell out of there and was gone. I don't think they ever collected the fine on *that* ship.

I took my general surgery board examinations while I was stationed in Alaska. I was fortunate that I got through them because I never had time to study and all I had was one book for review. After I took my written exam in Anchorage, I had to fly to San Francisco for the oral exam. My family came with me. After being isolated in the Aleutians for a year, we took time to travel together throughout California, going as far south as San Diego where we went to its famous zoo. Everyone had a great time. That trip turned out to be our one jaunt off the island in our two years there.

Once my years of service were completed, I had several job offers, but I decided to come back to Massachusetts to practice, since my wife and I both had family there. Because I had attended Holy Cross, I was familiar with the city of Worcester. I took what was supposed to be a temporary job at the nearby Fallon Clinic. I ended up working there for 27 years.

One of the patients I remember best was actually someone I had cared for when I was rotating through the heart service during my residency. Back then, open-heart procedures were still in their infancy and had a fairly high mortality rate. That was one of the rotations during which you practically lived at the hospital. If you were on the heart service as the senior resident, you were there 24/7. The only time you got home was when a patient died. Then there was no need to stay overnight.

This particular patient was an 18-year-old athlete with a bad congenital heart problem that had gone unrecognized. When he finally came in for surgery, it was probably too late. He looked like such a healthy, strapping young guy. But he died on the table. Everyone who had taken care of him felt badly.

But the next day, in the paper was a letter he had written prior to his surgery, almost foreseeing his own death. In the letter, he told his loved ones that he was going to miss them, but that they shouldn't feel badly. He also told the people who had taken care of him in the hospital not to be upset. As his surgeon, this letter was a real gift to me. He was a Catholic and maybe that had nothing to do with his letter, but he had a strong faith. I tear up even now when I think about him. The whole ordeal was such a moving experience and, ironically, it was the only time during that rotation that I ever got home. When I opened the door, my oldest boy, who was still pretty young, called out, "Hey, Daddy's home! Someone must've died!"

Sometimes bad events have silver linings. I've seen that so many times. You give a patient or a family bad news, "I can't do much for you," and watch how they react. Initially there's grief, but so often they suddenly get stronger, not only revealing the strength of the human spirit, but invariably their faith as well. During times like this, one can't help but marvel at the human race, how we've been given this gift of being able to support each other. Of all the things I've gotten out of practicing medicine, witnessing the way families strengthen each other and unify the human spirit is the one thing I'll remember most.

When I have bad news to deliver to a family, I've found that it doesn't take long to see who the spokesperson is, who the strong person is, and who the weak person is. I may speak to the weak person and comfort him first, because then the strong family members can follow my lead and continue to strengthen the weaker members. You've got to make eye contact, but sometimes it takes more. Sometimes the physician needs to put a hand on a shoulder or even give a hug. You've got to do what you can to establish direct contact and get them to trust you. Once you've established trust, the rest flows.

I stay away from blaming patients, families, and other physicians for someone's condition. There's no "Oh, she should have come in earlier for this." Most of the time, there really isn't one factor to blame, or the blame is shared. It's better if you stay away from blame.

I learned early on that it's good to share personally with patients. They will remember you not because you were able to cut and do something to fix them, but because you spent the time to talk to them and gave them support. Some surgeons don't make this kind of connection because they don't take the time to build trust between themselves and their patients. They're missing out on what's probably the nicest thing that can happen to a physician—getting that pat on the back. I've had patients, whom I no longer recognize, see me on the street and come over to give me a hug. I didn't get the hugs because of the surgery I performed, but because I talked to them and held their hands and got them through a rough period in their life. They always remember that.

Thank God, most surgeries are successful and people are grateful. It's always great to give somebody good news because that builds your ego. But because not every surgery is successful, you can't let your ego get the best of you. This is something that some surgeons never learn. The "God complex" is very common in the medical profession as well as in politics, sports, entertainment, and industry. But if you had to rank professions, according to their need to "play God," I think surgeons would be at the top of that list because they tend to have that type of personality. Several things contribute to this including the strenuous training program for surgery, which is similar to boot camp in the military. But in a way, surgeons are always in boot camp—going, going all the time. They are making decisions and sometimes life hangs in the balance. Sometimes the decision must be made rapidly; there is no time to waffle about it. When someone needs an operation, they need it now. Period. Do it.

Over the years, my family grew. We had three children of our own but became interested in adoption. One of the other surgeons we got to know in Massachusetts had adopted a child from Korea. We contacted the agency, which was located near Boston in

Newton. We looked at pictures of children waiting for a home. One photo jumped out at us, a picture of a brother and sister at an orphanage in Seoul.

"Oh!" said the social worker. "Are you interested in siblings?" Well, we had initially wanted to adopt just one child but these kids looked sad, so we said yes.

It didn't take long for the kids to arrive. At the time we adopted them, the boy was six and his sister was two. They turned out to be two of the nicest kids. Our daughter eventually graduated from the University of Massachusetts and is now a social worker in New Bedford, married and the mother of a cute little boy. Our son attended Worcester Polytechnic and became an engineer.

Not long after our first adoption, I got a call from an organization called Heal the Children, which was based in Washington state. They knew we had adopted two Korean children. "How did you hear about that?" I asked. "Well, we have a pipeline," they told me. They asked if I'd consider having some children come from Korea to have surgery. "Sure, why not?" I replied.

So we started getting Korean kids coming in for surgery. At first it was all heart procedures. Since UMass in Worcester hadn't yet developed a pediatric heart program, they went to Children's Hospital in Boston. At that time, hospitals donated a certain number of surgery slots for free care for international kids. We also developed connections with other humanitarian organizations that started sending us children for surgery.

The children would stay at our house while they were here in the United States. When they recovered, they went back to their native country. Over the years, 36 different surgical patients came to stay with us. Of these, we had two who died. The death of one of these patients, who was from Korea, upset my wife a lot because our children were from Korea. He was an older heart patient, in his late 20s, and because of his age and condition, he probably was not a great candidate for surgery. I think he had been cared for by a religious order in Korea because he had a tremendous faith. We have a little Crucifix at the bottom of the stairs at our house and every day he knelt before it and said prayers. We tried to keep him upbeat and active, but after the surgery he steadily deteriorated and eventually died.

So what do you do with a body from another country? He had family back in Korea, but transporting a body back there was not exactly the easiest thing in the world. It would involve a lengthy legal process. Fortunately I knew several undertakers, and one offered to finance a cremation. The urn with his ashes sat on our mantle for the longest time. It was driving my wife crazy because she had to look at it all the time. Finally, I found a Korean physician who was going back to visit his relatives. He agreed to take the urn in his carry-on luggage and deliver it to the young man's family. So at least we completed the circle and the young man was returned to his homeland. I heard that his family was very appreciative.

Another one of our very religious patients from Korea did much better after his surgery. He was in his 40s when he came. He was referred by a nun, Sr. Michaela, who worked with Heal the Children. After he returned home he called us every year on my birthday and my wife's birthday. The phone would ring—usually at 3:00 a.m. I never knew who was calling—him or one of my patients. But then I'd hear a voice say, "Hello, Fodder!" He spoke very little English but he would sing "Happy Birthday" or some little Korean song. Eventually after about ten years we stopped hearing from him. I think his heart disease finally caught up with him. But little things like his calls and all the Christmas cards we get from the children who stayed with us really touch me.

Along with a local priest and several parishioners at our parish, I founded a medical missions organization called CHANGE. We started out making trips to Guatemala, Nicaragua and Ecuador. We chose Central America because I had some familiarity with Spanish and because it was close enough so we could fly down and hit the ground running. I didn't go on every trip myself—I couldn't take that kind of time off—but I ran the program and established contacts in each of the countries. We kept sending supplies and teams down and occasionally brought a child up to the States for care.

As time went on I stopped doing overseas work and started doing local mission work. Although the need might not be as acute as in some of the poor countries we had served, there is still need here. In 1996, we started a free medical clinic at St. Anne's Church in Shrewsbury for people with no insurance. It was an ideal setting, since the parish already had a food bank and a thrift shop and was located on a bus route. People come from all over the area for services and the free clinic has grown to serve more than 90 people on one evening each week.

We have since started two more clinics that serve over 50 patients a week in Hispanic, Portuguese-speaking, and East African parts of the city. We have a fourth in the works, which will probably open in the spring in another needy section of Worcester where the population is mainly Vietnamese and Hispanic. We're expanding all the time because of the need.

At the clinics we provide primary care (including immunizations) as well as mental health care, and we have social workers who try to help our patients get insurance. We also try to get them the medications they need, but this can present problems because many younger physicians write prescriptions for expensive brand-name drugs that people can't afford. When this happens, patients will bring us their prescriptions and occasionally we can provide that drug for them. But if we can't, we try to direct them to an effective but less expensive alternative. Or we'll help them apply to a pharmaceutical company's patient assistance program, and if they meet the income requirements they may be able to receive the drug for free.

I put in a lot of hours at the clinics. We've never had a problem getting nurses to staff them, but we don't have as many doctors as I'd like. Our physicians include retired doctors, doctors who volunteer through St. Vincent Hospital, and a lot of foreign medical graduates who are doctors in their native countries but are not yet licensed to practice medicine in the United States. Some of them are very good, but I have to monitor them and sign off on what they do.

I'm a firm believer in the concept that faith evolves and must be nurtured throughout your lifetime. Though some elements of faith may be planted during childhood by your parents and through school, the seed of faith takes time to grow. The experiences of your life are a great influence on your faith. My own faith has been strengthened by the great faith I have seen in some of my patients. Being a witness to severe poverty also strengthens faith. For example, I remember being impressed by the fact that the children in Guatemala—a very Catholic country—had little in terms of material things, yet they were still happy, still smiling, still respectful, and still going to church on Sundays. Despite their poverty, they were very faithful to their families and to their religion.

There is an element of trust in any faith. With faith in God, you essentially have to put your life in God's hands. It's kind of like the faith you have in a doctor, particularly a surgeon who's going to have your life in his hands for a period of time. Typically, you've never met the surgeon before, but you need to have an operation.

This leaves a very short window of time to establish faith and trust that the surgeon is going to get you through the procedure.

Over time my life experience has strengthened my faith to the point where I don't need to waffle. I've thought through all the alternative explanations and now I have no question about my beliefs. I'm still an individualist. I don't rely on someone else to give me answers as I did in the past, when I relied on my teachers because they knew more about the faith than I did. My approach now to keeping my faith strong is a very practical one: I live it, every day.

I try to live my faith every day at work, but also at home. For example, several years after adopting the two children from Korea, my wife, Anne, and I were talking about how good our adoption experience had been and we began thinking that God was leading us to take in one more child. In the adoption magazines, we kept seeing this group of four siblings from Korea, cute as a button. They were in the magazine one year—and still in there the next year. The youngest was a boy aged one and a half and then there were three girls aged three, four, and six. Anne and I felt sorry for them but then we thought, "Oh God, how could we take *four*?" It would be a huge task; we already had five children. After talking it over, speaking with the social worker, and praying about the decision, we finally said, "Okay, let's do it."

The adoption process moved quickly and in less than three months, the four children arrived. They turned out to be a bit more work than even we had anticipated. The children arrived with heavy emotional baggage. The three girls had been especially traumatized, making it extremely difficult for them to bond with and to establish a trusting relationship with us. We consulted with psychiatrists and pediatricians, people we hoped were more knowledgeable about these problems than we were.

The girls were suffering from post-traumatic stress disorder and from the psychological effects of adoption. Their cultural background also affected their behavior. There was no easy solution and basically we had to learn along with the psychiatrists how to deal with the girls' problems. We were advised several times that the adoption had failed, that it was crazy to put ourselves and the rest of our family through this, and that we should send the kids back to Korea. For a while we anguished over what to do, but finally decided to stick it out, keep the children, and see what we could do to improve their lives.

We found some support groups that had just begun forming to help families who had adopted children from different countries. We had to travel to Boston to attend these evening group sessions, but it was good to hear from families who were going through similar problems with their kids. My wife and I used to joke that we'd drive the hour to Boston without saying much, but the ride home would be a non-stop debate about which approach we should use to help the kids.

We tried to help the children to maintain a sense of their Korean identity. We went with them to a local Korean Methodist church, enrolled them in Korean language classes, and sent them to a special culture camp. They never wanted to go, but we twisted their arms and they went. Ironically, now that they are adults, they want to learn about their heritage.

We got through some difficult times in their school-age years, but as teenagers it was worse. The children began reliving the trauma they'd known in Korea. That's not uncommon; it's the reason you see more suicide attempts, acting out, drugs, and promiscuity among such kids during their teen years. In addition, it was difficult for our kids to sort out the difference between the reality of their experiences and their fantasies about them. They also had to clarify their sense of identity and gain self-esteem in a foreign environment.

It took a while, but our adopted kids are now a lot more interested in their Korean heritage, after all those childhood years of wanting to be Americans. Two of them, in fact, have taken their Korean names in place of the names we gave them, which we think is good—we don't mind that at all. We want them to feel comfortable with themselves wherever they fit in. Then we'll feel our role as parents is complete.

Working long hours, I wasn't always there for Anne or for the kids. Medicine can be very demanding to the point of leading one to put work ahead of family and personal issues. I admire physicians who can successfully balance both. I could never say no and calling hours meant little when a patient was in great need. But we survived and worked with the kids on their problems, sometimes with professional help. Each has his or her own unique talent. The four adoptive siblings have creative talents from fashion design to writing to photography. We are proud of all of them. None of the children went into a career in medicine but I have no regrets. My eldest son came close; he is a biomedical engineer doing great research.

The youngest of the four Korean siblings, the boy, experienced trauma at a younger age than his sisters, and it was easier for him to develop a good relationship with us. He graduated from college with a degree in journalism and worked at a publishing house in New York City. He was the only one of our Korean children to develop a trusting relationship with another Korean. His girlfriend, who was also adopted from Korea, had an intense desire to travel to Korea to get back to her roots.

Anne and I and the kids all went to church together—we took up an entire pew. The adopted children were baptized and made their First Communion and Confirmation, but didn't adhere to any organized faith once they got out on their own. I think that's related to their inability to develop trust. It took years for them to find comfort in their Korean heritage. Their faith may develop in time as well. I know God loves us all and find comfort in remembering the parable of the Prodigal Son.

So now our story is up to nine kids. Number 10 came from Guatemala. She had come up here when she was seven years old for surgery, almost blind in one eye from glaucoma. She stayed with us while she was being treated, but then we lost touch with her for about a year. During that time she traveled illegally with her mother from Guatemala through Mexico to the U.S. One day out of the blue, she called to tell me that she was in California, that her eye hadn't been taken care of in a while, and that it hurt. So we brought her here, took care of her eye, and sent her back to California. Then she met a guy who got her pregnant and when her mother died, I got another call. She didn't have anybody in California whom she trusted. She was still only a teenager and was alone with a baby. "Okay," we said. "Come on back."

While she was living with us, she met a nice young man from Puerto Rico and they made plans to get married at our house on New Year's Eve. That evening, with a houseful of guests awaiting the ceremony, the minister failed to show up. We found out later that his flight to Massachusetts had been delayed and he had no way to contact us. After making last-minute phone calls to different ministers I knew from town, we finally found one who wasn't going out for New Year's Eve. She came over, and we had the ceremony.

This adoptive daughter lives not far away, in Worcester. She has four kids now, and although eventually she lost the sight in one eye and also suffers from diabetes, the glaucoma in her other eye is pretty well controlled.

Somewhere in there, we also took in a couple of rebellious sons of other doctors. I don't know what the family issues were—I guess it was just a phase of life they were going through—but when things got to the point that it was intolerable for them to remain with their parents, over they came to us. Fortunately they weren't both here at the same time! They each stayed with us maybe six or eight months, until things cooled off at home. Now both of them are college graduates with families and are doing well.

So that completes our family tree: ten kids (three of our own, two from Korea, then four from Korea, and finally one from Guatemala), thirteen grandchildren, and a dog!

Life hasn't been easy. Anne and I have had our ups and downs. We've been married nearly 48 years and I can't say every one of them was smooth. We've argued many a time, but mostly because our kids were playing one of us against the other. But ironically, it was after the last kid left home that we went through an especially difficult time. I thought, "Great! Finally—peace!" But my wife had the opposite reaction and went into a deep depression. She had done so much for the kids and suddenly she felt her life was over. Boy, that was a rough few months, but we got through it. Now our problems are just some minor health issues, arthritis and the surgeries involved with that—nothing life-threatening. We push each other to stay active, both mentally and physically, and we help each other stay out of trouble. I think that sometimes you need someone to tell you, "You're an idiot! Don't let your ego get the best of you!" That's good, because sometimes you don't recognize it yourself.

Our life has always been centered on actively living our faith in our daily lives. Our relationship with a church community has been a little more uneven. We attended St. Mary's Church when the kids were in the parish school, and we remained involved in parish life until the kids were finally out of school and out of the house. Then I got involved with St. Anne's Church—that was 13 years ago. St Anne's is a different kind of parish. There's no school. Their mission and ministry is helping people through human services, especially now with the health clinic.

You know, I have no real regrets. There have been a lot of ups and downs in our lives, but the ups are still way ahead of the downs. There's always a silver lining somewhere if you look for it. I tell people that no matter what happens or how bad it seems, if you think about your problems, reflect on them, give it a little time and don't act rashly, you'll probably find there's a reason behind what happened and that with faith some good will come out of it.

I'll give you an example of how that advice helped me. About 10 years ago, after I had worked for 27 years at the Fallon Clinic, I was let go. Medicine was changing; the computer era began. The clinic started using electronic medical records, and in the operating room, the focus was shifting to laparoscopic surgery. Some of us who were a little resistant to these changes had been there a long time and had built up pretty decent pensions. The administration probably thought, "Let's get rid of a few older doctors and save some money. Then we'll hire young new physicians who are up on the newest technology." So a few of us were let go.

The way they did it was not acceptable to me. My work there had been my life; all my friends were there. A year earlier they had cut my salary because I was giving free care to patients who needed it. The notice that I was being let go came at the end of the day on a Friday. The reason they cited was "poor patient care." I came home and told Anne and we cried together. We kept telling each other our usual philosophy, that something good was going to come out of this, even though we couldn't see any good at the time.

Well, the phone started ringing the next day. Word of my dismissal had gotten out to some of my patients and I'd taken care of a lot of patients over the years. Patients called saying that they'd heard the news and were offering to start a petition to have me reinstated. They also notified a reporter from the *Telegram & Gazette*, our local newspaper, and the next day she came to interview me. I showed her the documents about my salary cut and my letter of dismissal. Sure enough, a day later, I was on the front page of the paper, picture and all. The paper received letters about the story and the reporter got email responses from readers, prompting her to write another piece about it. The publicity didn't exactly put the Fallon Clinic in a good light.

The silver lining part—the reason why I'm telling this story—was that I got a phone call from another doctor here in town, who owned the building where his practice was located. He offered me space for minimal rent to start a practice in his building. "Come on down and practice for as long was you want," he told me.

That was 10 years ago. I had to go through a lot of red tape to get re-credentialed as an individual rather than as a group provider. But since then, I've developed a nice little practice that has allowed me to do a lot of the good things I like to do, such as teaching and giving care to patients in the free clinics. The practice also allows me to come home and sleep at night without a lot of headaches. I exercise more and I even have time to teach exercise classes. I don't do surgery anymore—the malpractice insurance would be prohibitively expensive—but I'm earning enough so that Anne and I can get along without dipping into our nest egg.

The other silver lining was that I had the rare opportunity to have my "obituary" written when I was 60 years old and I got to read it myself! Don't laugh—I'm serious. I've saved the pack of letters that were sent to me by patients who told me how wonderful our interactions had been, telling me that what had happened was terrible and that they were really going to miss me. They were the kind of letters that most of us never get to see in this life. What a twist of fate! I received "bad news" and my patients supported me and restored my self-esteem and faith!

Wow, what a boost that was for me. Here I'd been killing myself, doing 650 cases a year—that's a lot of surgery—and being on call every other night. Now that I look back on it, being let go probably happened at an opportune time. I wish it had happened a few years later and it bothered me for a little while, especially the reason given for letting me go, that they didn't like the way I'd been practicing medicine. But in the long run, wounds heal and there's always a reason for things—always that silver lining.

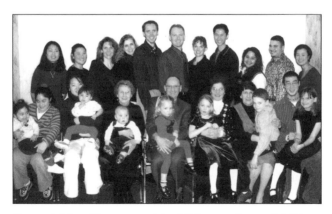

Dr. and Mrs. Clermont with children and grandchildren

— *Ad Majorem Dei Gloriam* —

8

Dr. John Donovan

FROM PRIEST TO PEDIATRICIAN

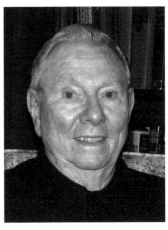

I didn't start out to be a doctor. I started by spending five years in the seminary studying to become a priest, and voluntarily left when I realized that my vocation lay elsewhere. When I left, the last thing Monsignor Reilly, our dean of discipline, said to me was "John, now you can go out with girls!" But the "girl thing" wasn't what compelled me to leave. It was the knowledge that if I became a priest, I couldn't have a family of my own. Since I've always loved children, I guess it only stands to reason that I'd become a pediatrician, and for 47 years, that's what I was.

As a child, I had a good solid Catholic upbringing. My dad was Catholic and my mother converted to the Faith when she married him. Her conversion prompted a rift with her sister. The two of them were estranged for quite a while because of the conversion. Dad was a grocer who ran a liquor store as part of his business. I didn't see much of him as a kid; he was always down at the store working.

My mother was a saint—she lived a beautiful life and prayed constantly. She made sure I attended Mass and went to Confession regularly. She and my father sent me to parochial school and to St. John's Catholic High School for boys. At our parish church I was an altar server. My mother was always after me to be a good boy. If I ever said a bad word or told the slightest hint of a lie, she would reprimand me for it. Back then, it was expected by our parents that we would practice our faith.

I was something of a troublemaker at St. John's. Perhaps my red hair gave me my temper. I could raise the *divil* if my temper got away from me. I used to wiggle my ears (I still can), which would make everyone sitting behind me laugh. Then I'd pretend I didn't know what was going on. I must have driven my teachers crazy, but I did well enough in my studies to be the valedictorian of our class.

Maybe my academic achievements prompted our parish priest to urge me to enter the seminary. I had no strong desire of my own to enter the priesthood, but this priest, along with my mother, seemed convinced that it was the right thing for me to do. My mentor, Brother Walston, shared that opinion too. He had taken me under his wing in high school, talking with me about my interests. He even outfitted me with hockey gear when my dad was struggling financially. I think he envisioned me as a priest or a teaching brother like himself. In the end I wound up attending St. John's Seminary in Brighton.

I was in the seminary from 1945 to 1950, and, to tell the truth, I relished my years there. I met some wonderful guys, and the bunch of us became like brothers. We were so close and we did everything together. We studied hard, did all kinds of athletics, and in the summers went together to the seminary camp at Lake Winnipesaukee in New Hampshire. In fact, our bond was so strong that at one point, our teachers told us to break up the clique.

In the seminary we were pretty isolated from the rest of the world. No television, no newspapers, no radio. I used to send my dirty laundry home to Marlborough, and my mother would send it back clean, folded and wrapped up in the latest edition of the local paper. So I'd get some news, along with my clean laundry. She'd usually add some cookies or other treat.

And we got into some *divilment* of our own there too. One day we were calmly and quietly taking our showers—it was against the rules to talk. Each shower stall had a bucket and my friend Louie filled his full of ice-cold water and tossed it over the stall divider onto me. I filled my own bucket with cold water to retaliate, but couldn't see Louie frantically shaking his head, mouthing the word "Nooooo!" I stood on the shower bench and reached over the divider to toss the water. It splashed all over Monsignor Reilly, the dean of discipline, who'd been roaming the corridors and had come to investigate the noise. He glared at me over his eyeglasses. "I'll see you in my office when you're finished here," he told me sternly. I don't remember my punishment, but I think the monsignor knew it was innocent tomfoolery on our part.

But despite all the camaraderie, I began to feel very unhappy in the seminary. I found that I was reading more of Carl Sandburg's

Life of Lincoln than of *Summa Theologica*. I started thinking more about what was going to happen when I finished my studies. I began to see that I was only staying for the sense of brotherhood and that I had entered the seminary because I felt pushed by my pastor and my mother. But although I realized I didn't have a vocation to the priesthood, I hated the thought of leaving my "brothers."

Instead of studying, I spent a lot of time in the chapel late at night, praying to the good Lord to tell me what to do. I was praying so much at night that I started falling asleep during morning prayers with my class. Monsignor Reilly, who was a peach of a man despite his stern demeanor, knew how I was feeling. Finally, after a heart-to-heart talk with him, he agreed that I should take a break, and sent me off with his blessing.

I took the bus home from Brighton and showed up at my doorstep, suitcase in hand. It was so hard to break the news to my mother. She couldn't imagine anything greater than having a son become a priest. She was bitterly disappointed that I'd left. She cried for a long, long time. In fact, it got so bad that I had to go to live for a while with my sister in North Attleboro, because every time my mother saw me, she'd burst into tears. My dad, on the other hand, didn't mind as much. Since I was his only son, I think he had seen the end of the Donovan line when I entered the seminary. But he had gotten to love all the guys in my class as much as I did and he enjoyed having them come over for visits, when they'd practically take over our little house.

Louie, my partner in "crime," turned into a wonderful priest. He was a rogue, but he was a love. He was ordained for service in Vermont, where he built a camp for handicapped and autistic children, and a chapel to our Lady of the Snows to serve the skiers. But he kept his *divilish* streak. Whenever someone asked him, "Father Louie, why didn't you marry some girl instead of becoming a priest?" his eyes would twinkle and he'd answer, "If I'd married one, twenty would have committed suicide."

So one week I left the seminary and the next week I joined the U.S. Air Force. I went down to the recruiting station in Boston, where I got a warm welcome. "We always like volunteers," the recruiter told me. "What kind of education do you have?" I told him I'd spent five years earning a degree in philosophy, studying to be a Catholic priest. "Well," he replied, "if you want to change your religion, we can make you a captain right now as a chaplain."

"No, thanks," I answered. "I'll take my chances in Officer Training School."

My seminary training served me well and I breezed right through training for the Air Force. My classmates used to ask me, "How can you take this so easily?" Since the rules and regulations in the seminary had seemed much stricter to me, I didn't mind the discipline and what's more, I had gotten my temper under control in the seminary. I ended up graduating with distinction and becoming a training officer. I served for three years at Lackland Air Force Base during the Korean War, after which I was eligible for release. That's when my thoughts turned to medicine.

I had left the seminary, but I still wanted to do something worthwhile. My grandfather had been a physician so I thought I'd try medicine, but I knew it wouldn't be easy because I didn't have enough science credits from my curriculum at the seminary. I spent two years at Boston College getting caught up. And then I had a little trouble getting into Tufts Medical School. When I got my letter of rejection I spoke with Fr. Walsh, my mentor at B.C. He called Tufts and arranged for a special interview with the admissions office. They asked why I had decided to leave the seminary and become a doctor. I told them I thought a good way to get to a person's spiritual life was to take care of the person's physical well-being. I guess they liked that answer because they finally admitted me.

I met my future wife Ellie at the wedding of a mutual friend. She very nearly didn't go, because she had been on late duty at her nursing job that day. But her aunt talked her into going, hinting that she "might meet someone." We dated for three years before we got married in 1956, during my second year of med school. One of the priests with whom I had studied in the seminary celebrated our Nuptial Mass. Ellie came back from the honeymoon pregnant with our first child. I still remember going down to my dad's liquor store to tell him of his first grandchild's birth. Dad himself never drank, but that night he instructed his employee to get down the best bottle of whiskey in the store. He proclaimed, "We're all going to have a drink to John Henry Donovan III."

While I was in medical school at Tufts, Ellie and I lived in Charlestown, just below the Bunker Hill Monument. One of the priests who had attended the seminary with me became the pastor of our parish. When he found out that "Red Jack" Donovan was now one of his parishioners, guess who had to sing the psalms at the Easter Vigil, in Latin, dressed up in cassock, surplice, the whole kit and caboodle! After it was over, a little old lady came up to Ellie and remarked, "I didn't know you were married to a priest!"

I finished med school at age 33 and did my internship and pediatric residency at St. Vincent Hospital in Worcester. Pediatrics was perfect for me because I loved kids. Since our family was growing rapidly, I needed to get out into practice to earn an income. And so I opened an office in the town of Shrewsbury. I was fortunate that a couple of grand pediatricians in Worcester encouraged their patients from Shrewsbury to transfer to my office. I was accepted into the medical community here with no ifs, ands or buts. Ellie and I put down roots in Shrewsbury and joined St. Mary's Church, which is still our parish home. We tried to raise our own children with the same strong faith that our parents had given us.

Goodness knows I needed my faith every day in my work with patients. Early in my practice I had a little patient who was severely retarded and very sick. There didn't seem to be much hope for him so I spoke with his parents about whether they wanted a do-not-resuscitate order, but they couldn't reach a decision. One day when the sick child was brought to the hospital, he went into respiratory distress and someone resuscitated him. I remember asking God why he had to keep on suffering. The child ended up on a breathing apparatus in the ICU at St. Vincent Hospital. I prayed and prayed for guidance and when I called his parents his mother told me, "Do whatever you think is necessary." All the way to the hospital I prayed, "Please, Lord, help me to do the right thing."

When I got there I told the nurses that we would remove the respirator. And that's what we did. But I learned that night that I couldn't play God because, lo and behold, the patient started breathing on his own. We kept him in the ICU for a few days and then sent him home. He lived for a few more days, still breathing on his own, and finally died peacefully in his sleep at home.

I could almost hear God telling me, "John Henry, you think you're the good Lord but you don't rule life and death. The good Lord is running life and death, not you." That night I learned a profound lesson and I'm very thankful that I learned it early on. Medicine is a humbling profession. I realized that I'm just an instrument in the hands of the Holy Spirit—the Holy Spirit is the one running the show. It still brings tears to my eyes to think about it. If you can't feel that way about your patients, you're a cold cucumber.

In those days I used to go out on a lot of house calls and, of course, weekends and nights I was on call. When that happened, the phone would ring at the house as well as at the office. One weekend alone I fielded 176 phone calls. Some of the calls were just hilarious in retrospect although at 3:00 a.m. they were more annoying than funny.

"Dr. Donovan," said one voice in the middle of the night, "Pudgie won't take his heartworm pill." "I'm sorry, ma'am," I answered, "but I'm Dr. Donovan, the pediatrician, not Dr. Donovan the vet."

Another 3:00 a.m. caller was frantic, telling me that I had to come over right away. "My daughter's gone blind!" he shrieked into the phone. "She's screaming and crying that she can't see!" "Could you do me a favor?" I asked, with all the patience I could muster. "Could you please go to her room and turn on the light?" I could hear his footsteps as he put down the phone and walked down the hallway to the bedroom. A minute later he was back on the phone. "Oh, my goodness," he said, embarrassment in his voice. "I'm sorry, doc."

But I think the prize for late-night wake-up calls went to the woman who demanded, "Doctor, I need you to tell me how to use a rectal thermometer." Ellie, as usual, had been awakened by the call and had heard the question. She clutched my arm. "Don't you *dare* tell her what you're thinking," she warned me. I didn't. But I did give the patient clinical instructions. Talk about laughing after I hung up on that one!

So much has changed for the better in medicine since my practice began back in the 1960's. I remember my first leukemia patient. His mother had brought him along to his brother's appointment, but I kept looking at him, not at the patient, because something didn't seem right. I asked his mother if I could examine him first. I saw that he had little petechiae, tiny blood hemorrhages, on his skin along with swelling of the lymph glands. His liver, his spleen, and every lymph node in his body were swollen.

"Please sit down," I told his mother. "You've got to take him to the hospital right away. He's got leukemia." Within the hour the hematologist at the hospital confirmed my diagnosis. The little boy lasted only a few months. Today, with the new treatments that are available, a high percent of leukemia patients go into remission.

One night I was called to the emergency room for a patient who was celebrating his first birthday. His father had brought him in with a temperature of 105 degrees and he was hoping that he would be able to take the child home for his birthday party. But he was much too sick to be sent home. I carried the baby up to the pediatric ward myself and by the time we got to the elevator he had broken out with petechiae. He had meningococcal meningitis. It's a disease that can quickly become deadly. Shortly after we got up to the ward, the child stopped breathing. I worked on that baby for a long time, trying to revive him, giving him mouth-to-mouth resuscitation; I didn't care whether I got the disease as a result. But despite all my efforts, the little boy died on his first birthday. It broke my heart. The two of us, the father and I, sat down and talked and cried together.

Another patient who lived near us came into the office with a high fever. She turned out to have Reye's syndrome. I sent her from the office right to the hospital where they packed her in ice but she went into a seizure that lasted, I don't know how long. We called the Cleveland Clinic that night and asked their advice, which was to give a total exchange transfusion. So we began processing eight units of blood for the procedure but she died before we could begin.

Her dad and I cried together and then I came home, sat down, and cried with Ellie. All I could think of was how I'd feel if I lost my own daughter to that kind of disease. Her father had brought her in to my office, and within 12 hours she was gone. Outcomes like that used to make me turn to the good Lord, to try to help parents get through their loss, rather than pass it off as just another case. And I needed the strength to get through the losses myself.

Our family grew to include seven children and my practice became a family affair. Ellie eventually joined me in the office—I think she figured it was the only way she'd get to see me, with the hours I had to keep. My patients called her "Mrs. Dr. Donovan." Because she had been the head nurse of a newborn nursery department before we were married, I learned more from her about the care of premature babies than I'd ever learned in med school. Ellie Donovan knew all the ins and outs, all the tricks of the trade. As each of our five girls reached high school age they also came to work at the office and in this way found out how much work the old man had to do!

The work was a lot of fun, but there were lots of tears too. If I hadn't had the good Lord and the Holy Spirit on my shoulder I don't think I could have done it. And I certainly couldn't have managed without Ellie's support. She kept me sane and she did a wonderful job raising our seven children, to a large extent on her own.

Sometimes I'd struggle for a diagnosis. I don't know that I'd call it "enlightenment" when the answer materialized. But when it finally came into my head I'd always say, "Thank you, Lord." One case that I just prayed and prayed about involved a little baby whose mother kept bringing him into my office with persistent high temperatures. I couldn't find a thing wrong with him apart from the fever; he always looked well although he had unusually dry skin.

Well, on one of my days off, a friend and I were playing golf at Pleasant Valley and we were sweating like mad because of the heat. As I was getting ready to go up for my shot, I suddenly threw my golf club into the air and shouted, "I know what the kid's got!" My golf partner looked at me strangely and asked, "What are you doing?"

"I know what the kid's got," I repeated. "The Holy Spirit told me." The good Lord had tapped me on the shoulder and told me, "He doesn't sweat." The boy had a rare disease called anhydrotic ectodermal dysplasia—a lack of sweat glands over the entire body. He was unable to regulate his body temperature. I went home and got out my medical books and discovered he was a textbook case.

Another time, a mother called me in the early morning hours about her son. He had gone to the emergency room with a severe migraine but the staff there had failed to find anything and had sent him home. I told the mother to bring him into the office first thing in the morning. The Holy Spirit tapped me on the shoulder and prompted me to look into the boy's eyes—which the emergency room staff had not done. When I did, it became immediately clear that he had a brain tumor. He went into surgery the next day and it was successfully removed. Today he's raising a family of six children.

I tried to keep my trust centered on the good Lord. I loved my practice, but we were busy, busy, busy all the time. Sometimes it got so that you'd wish you could go and hide. When I was tired and weary I used to pray, "Dear God, please help me be patient with the patients." You read so much about people complaining over the long wait to see the doctor, but once people got in to see me, I'd give them the full time they needed to be examined. I only remember one exception when a lady stormed out because she'd been waiting too long.

And sometimes tensions rose among the children. One time I had to go out into the waiting room after a fight broke out. One child had hit another over the head with a metal toy and I had to stitch up the victim! We got rid of the metal toys in pretty short order.

The good Lord did give me a vacation once, in the dead of winter when it was 18 degrees below zero. Ellie had baked two cherry pies for the women's guild at church, and I'd packed them into the car to deliver them. Then the phone rang. One of my patients was having a convulsion and I needed to get to the ER. As I tried to back the car out, it got stuck in a snowdrift. As I got out to try to push it free, I hit a patch of bare ice, slid, and broke my ankle.

Ellie was in the house with the kids but one of my sons heard me screaming. Ellie called for help and before long the fire department, the police, and the ambulance arrived. But they were held at bay by Kerry—my big black Lab, my guardian—who wouldn't let them near me. Finally, Ellie came out and opened the car door. The dog promptly jumped in—and sat down on her pies!

Meanwhile, I was numb with the cold, lying there on the driveway, but the firemen, police, and ambulance driver were in a great mood. Because I took care of all their kids, it was like old home week, right there in my driveway. Finally, they hauled me off in the ambulance, but they were having such a good time telling stories that they drove right by St. Vincent Hospital and into the next town before they realized they had to turn around.

When I finally got to the ER, since I was a staff member at the hospital, they called for the chief of anesthesia to come in. The first thing he did was take a pair of scissors and cut the pant leg off of my brand-new suit, right along the leg, not in the seam, where it could be repaired. They gave me a spinal and it didn't take too long for them to manipulate and reset my ankle. That night marked the start of my forced vacation.

I saw patients at four different hospitals in Worcester. At one I became the head of pediatrics. Since there were no interns, I spent a lot of time down there, doing spinal taps and IVs. I vividly recall the day there was a big staff meeting to discuss the possibility of performing abortions in the OB department. The discussion reignited my latent Irish temper and a verbal volcanic eruption ensued. Ice water and cool heads were necessary to extinguish the flames. The subject was tabled—and never brought up again.

In addition to my office practice and work at the hospital, I also served 27 years as the physician for the schools in Shrewsbury. During that time, the head of the Catholic school asked me to do a presentation on sex education for the fifth and sixth grade boys. At that age they were really more interested in what would happen if a baseball or a hockey puck hit them in the private area. But I tried to teach them the basics of anatomy and describe, quietly and reverently, the process of how the sperm unites with the egg.

"And then...BOOM!" I would shout. "Now there's another person, just like each one of you!" That explosion in my voice really made them all sit up and pay attention! I wanted them to realize what a wonderful thing was happening in a way that would make them remember it. It got back to me later that the boys were going around at recess in the playground shouting, "BOOM! BOOM!"

I tried to help my patients learn to respect their bodies as they grew. We had been brought up learning that our bodies are temples of the Holy Spirit, and should be treated as such and should never be debased or used for anything that's wrong. That's the kind of information I'd try to give the kids.

I had a little trick that I used to help kids feel good when they had to get a shot. I'd take the needle out quickly and would secretly bend the tip before I showed it to them. Then I'd say, "Look what beautiful big muscles you have! Look how strong you are!" Their eyes would get wide and they'd ask, "I did that?" and their tears would go right away. After I'd been in practice for a long time and started getting second-generation patients, one of my former patients brought his son in for a shot. When he saw me bend the needle he said, "Oh, no! I always thought that really was my muscles that did that!" I think he was disappointed that I'd shown him the secret.

I wasn't afraid to bring morality into my practice. I know that a lot of pediatricians have told me that they never taught their patients morality, but I definitely did. I never tried to convert anybody, but just a little word here and there can make a difference, especially with teens. I never talked down to my patients—never, never, never. But I might try to help them see a different side of certain problems. It was never any holier-than-thou business, just an attempt to instill a little common sense and decency, a little ethics.

I tried to encourage my little patients to listen to, love and obey their parents. If a boy was sassy to his mom, I would say sternly, "Don't you talk to your mother that way! You need to respect your mother. She's a model for you." Discipline had been a part of my upbringing and I wanted them to be disciplined properly. I could get very stern if I needed to make my point.

As kids get older, of course, the issues change. One father brought in his lovely 13-year-old daughter. She seemed very nervous and worried, and after I talked to her, it came out that she had kissed a boy and was worried that she was pregnant as a result. So I went through the entire "talk" about how kissing doesn't produce pregnancy. But I also emphasized that she should love and respect her body and refrain from the act that *would* produce pregnancy. I think maybe her father hadn't been able to bring himself to have this talk with her himself. In any case, she left my office with a smile on her face.

Occasionally, young girls would come in with tattoos and pierced body parts such as the tongue, lips, nose, and navel. Without reprimanding them, I cautioned these girls on the potential medical complications of these artistic expressions, and exhorted them to think long and hard before getting any more because, in later years, they might possibly regret those choices.

In the seminary, our teachers tried to help us become humble, hardworking souls; humility was the greatest virtue that they tried to instill in us. One of my favorite sayings is "Humility is truth." You have to accept who you are in the sight of God and work from there. I tried to bring that philosophy into my medical practice. I hate the idea of a doctor being a snob, looking down on people. You've got to treat people the way you want people to treat you. In our office we were just a happy family. None of us felt we were better than anyone else.

Over the years we had many patients and parents who enriched and inspired our own faith. Amy was one such patient. I was called to attend when this lovely little redhead was born by Caesarian section. I took care of her for her entire life. One day she came in with a sore hip; it turned out to be due to cancer, a neuroblastoma. We sent her out to Cleveland for a bone marrow transplant, but at only 16 years old, she died. Ellie and I attended her funeral service. Amy and her parents had such courage, even in the face of death.

Another little girl was Angela. She was a beautiful child with severe problems including a huge hemangioma occupying most of her brain. Unable to speak or do anything for herself, she could only smile and follow her parents with her eyes. Yet her parents were the happiest couple and very accepting of Angela's situation. They were determined to do the best they could to take care of her, accepting the fact that they had received this little soul from God. They treated her as an angel. We learned to do so as well. We relished seeing them when they came in, because they were always upbeat. They never complained, despite the fact that they had to do every single little thing for this girl. They also had a son, who was perfectly normal, and they taught him how to love too. He loved his sister, no matter how incapable she was of doing anything but returning that love with a smile.

We had other patients with special needs, suffering from various ailments. One father carried his little girl around with him everywhere and made special chairs for her. She had severe cerebral palsy and couldn't walk. You could see the love he had for his daughter, and she would look at him and smile that smile that was just for him. Another of my little patients, a girl with Down syndrome, used to call me "Dr. Dumbumbum." She'd hug and kiss me when she came in and I always felt good when I saw her. But whether a child like this responded to us or not, we saw him or her as a little person whom God had entrusted to their parents. We recognized that we had to take care of them like their parents did. The parents' example just strengthened our desire to treat everyone like that, like angels in our office.

Occasionally we'd meet with parents at a patient's home, to talk about the care of their special-needs child. I loved those families. They were the epitome of patience, and they gave me the desire to be more patient myself. We learned so much from those parents whose children were dealing with difficult physical and mental problems. It would make me go to my books and study a bit more on how to handle the ailments they faced. It made us work harder and better to assist them with treatments. We worked our souls out trying to find things that would help ease the burden for them. And it made us more humble and more grateful for the blessings of our own children's good health.

We too got a taste of the fears that parents experience. When our second son Dan, 10 months old, developed a fever, I took a look at him and noticed that he had no femoral pulses. "Ellie, grab my stethoscope!" I cried somewhat gruffly. I listened and heard a loud murmur. We took him to the hospital, where Dr. Stan, a close friend and cardiology resident, confirmed that Dan had a congenital heart defect. He had a coarctation of the aorta and patent ductus arteriosus. I was an intern there at the time so the news spread like wildfire throughout the hospital and beyond. Everyone was concerned about our son.

Once he was 10 years old and had grown a bit, Dan had corrective surgery at Massachusetts General Hospital. On the day of the operation, while he was on the operating table, I went up to the pediatric ward. To keep myself busy, I spent those tense hours wheeling kids around the ward in little carts. They were late finishing up the surgery and I was a wreck. I had a million worries going though my mind. But when the surgeon came out, he told me Dan had lost only one ounce of blood. He has a scar from the front of his torso to his back, but today he's a paramedic and a big, husky, handsome-looking fellow with three kids.

Now we're dealing with another medical crisis in our family. Six years ago our daughter Ellen, a non-smoker and married with two children, was diagnosed with lung cancer. She underwent surgery, radiation and chemotherapy at Dana-Farber Cancer Center in Boston, a most capable, competent and compassionate facility. She had good results for years. But last year a recurrence of the tumor was found and Ellen is now receiving a special oral medication attacking only the specific lung cancer cells. Everyone is praying for good results again. Please God![32]

We've all had our struggles, but now that I'm retired, I have plenty of time to spend with our seven kids and the thirteen grandchildren. To this day, former patients will come up to me in the store when we're out shopping and ask, "Dr. Donovan, don't you remember me?" Sometimes I have to admit, "Not with that beard, I don't!" Sometimes I like to embarrass them and say, "If you bared your bottom I'd probably remember you," because I gave so many shots over the years.

We're still busy with our parish, where I am now a lector as well as a Eucharistic minister. I've never seen religious duties as a chore, but rather I consider it a privilege to distribute the Body and Blood of Christ to my fellow parishioners. Before I retired, I couldn't commit to doing a lot of things. Medicine was my master, so to speak, because I'd get called out at all hours. Now I'm enjoying the chance to focus more on our family and our church.

---

32. Ellen Donovan Samia died in peace April 5, 2010 (Editor's note).

Whether we're called to the religious life or to the married life, we're all put on this earth to work hard and to gain heaven. Ellie and I have tried in our vocation to do the best we could in the sight of the good Lord and to serve as models for our children and grandchildren. We've tried to show them how to do what's right with God and His Church, not by lecturing but by example. We've tried to live good, holy lives and still be down-to-earth people. I think Ellie's been a better example than I've been—she truly is my much better half.

My time in the seminary has proven to be beneficial for life as a pediatrician. Going from almost-priest to full-fledged physician has enabled me to approach medical and spiritual problems with a clearer vision. It has also helped me realize that all my little patients and their parents are special in God's eyes, thereby deserving of the best possible care. I have mentioned only a few of the incidents that have happened during many years of practice. To describe them all would be a monumental undertaking. In a lifetime a pediatrician sees thousands of children with countless different problems. What I learned in seminary I have found helpful over the years as a pediatrician—hard work and perseverance, coupled with prayer and trust in God, the Author of life.

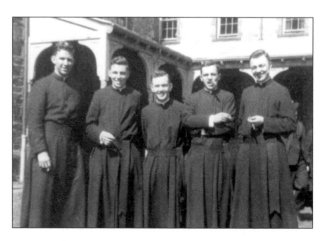

May 7, 1948. St. John Seminary.
Louis, John Donovan, Eddie, Frank, and Dick.

— Ad Majorem Dei Gloriam —

9

Dr. Mark Rollo

ABOUT MY FATHER'S BUSINESS

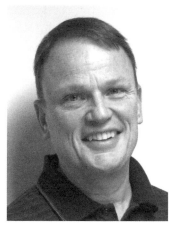

I was born in Boston. My first home there was in an Italian prisoner-of-war detention camp. You probably never knew such a thing existed in Boston—or even the United States—did you? It was established during World War II.[33] After the war it was converted into low-income housing.

My father was a surgeon. He was born in Fitchburg, Massachusetts. After receiving his medical degree at Indiana Medical School, he came back east to do his surgical residency at St. Elizabeth's Medical Center in Boston. Back in those days, residents really were residents—they pretty much lived in the hospital. They were on call every other night; they'd work 36 hours, go home for 12 hours, work 36, and go home for 12. My father was paid $25 a month, but he could eat his meals at the hospital. Surgeons were back then—and still are today—kind of macho people. Rather than complain about the long hours, they used to say that the only bad thing about being on call every other night was that they'd miss half the interesting cases.

My parents were very Catholic and very traditional. We never missed Mass on Sundays and holy days. My brothers and I were altar boys and since this was pre-Vatican II, we had to learn the Latin Mass. I certainly valued my faith at that time, but there was a sense of "this is what you do." It was simply a part of my life. I was in public elementary school, so I went to weekly CCD classes, but I don't have very fond memories of them. I don't think they made much of an impact on me.

---

33. During World War II the U.S. government forcibly relocated and detained some 120,000 Italian, German, and Japanese Americans in War Relocation Camps. The facility in East Boston was an Immigration Detention Station and was used to detain foreign nationals considered "potentially dangerous" who were later moved to one of the internment camps.

Back then religious education consisted of memorizing the Catechism. The nun told you to stand up and recite the relevant questions and answers. You hoped you'd get called last, because after everyone else had recited the answer, you'd know it!

When I was two years old we left the "prison camp" housing in Boston and moved to Washington state. My father had been drafted to serve in the Korean War. He was sent to Korea to serve with a M.A.S.H. unit. When he returned, we moved back to Massachusetts and ultimately to my father's hometown of Fitchburg, where I grew up. There were six of us siblings in all, five boys and a girl. I'm the second oldest; two of my brothers are also docs. My older brother, John, is a pathologist in St. Louis, and my younger brother Frank is an anesthesiologist in upstate New York. He's already semi-retired, because he got involved with online securities trading. They say that anesthesia is one of those specialties that involves hours of boredom and moments of terror when something goes wrong. It can be pretty stressful—but so can day trading, I guess.

Not only did my father encourage us to go into medicine, it was almost a foregone conclusion. He had our whole education mapped out: We would go to Notre Dame High School, the Catholic boys' high school in Fitchburg, where the Brothers of the Sacred Heart taught; then we'd go to the College of the Holy Cross, where my father had gone; and then on to medical school. That part was sort of optional—the selection of a medical school was left up to us.

My brothers John and Frank did it the conventional way. I took a more unconventional route—my grades weren't that good, and I wasn't sure I wanted to go into medicine anyway. I was a psychology/pre-med major at Holy Cross but toward the end of my time there I got interested in teaching. I enjoyed student teaching psychology and sociology at Doherty High School in Worcester. The kids, mostly juniors and seniors, were nice and were reasonably well behaved.

My wife, Annette, is also from Fitchburg. While I was attending Notre Dame High School, she was attending our "sister school," Holy Family, just over the hill. We met at one of the joint dances that the schools had together. She was a year behind me, and she actually dated one of my friends first. Then I went away to Holy Cross, but when I came back home, I discovered that she wasn't dating anybody.

If we were getting to know each other today, I'd probably email or call her on my cell phone. But I drove over to her house one Friday night around 9 o'clock. When I think back on it now, I must have startled her, knocking on her door at that hour. She came to the door and I said, "Hey! You want to go bowling?" She stammered, "Um, um....okay." So the next night, we went bowling. The bowling alley where we had our first date was right next door to my current office. Isn't that ironic? Annette and I had a long courtship, dating all through college, but early on we knew we were meant for each other. Almost every weekend I would use my "educated thumb" to travel to be with her.

After I graduated from Holy Cross, I decided to get a master's degree in education at the University of Massachusetts. I taught science to junior high school kids as a student teacher. But really, it was mostly just crowd control. I realized, "No, I don't think I want to do this after all." So I went back to school and in 1976 got my master's degree in social work from Boston College.

From there, I went to work at Northampton State Hospital in western Massachusetts, which has since closed down. Northampton State was a hospital for emotionally disturbed adults, most of whom were chronically sick and institutionalized. At the time I was there, in the 1970s, the state mental hospitals were going through a deinstitutionalization process. It was terrible. I'm sure there were some good intentions involved. But there were also many people trying to make a name for themselves by getting people out of the hospitals. These people who wanted to close the hospitals weren't the ones actually responsible for the patients' care. So they discharged a lot of people who had no skills and were unable to take care of themselves. As a result, instead of patients rocking in the corner of an institution and being cared for, they ended up homeless, sitting on a street corner rocking, and having people take advantage of them.

In some cases the deinstitutionalization process worked out well. People who had some skills were able to make the transition. But it was unrealistic to expect people who'd been in an institution for 10 years and had no social skills at all to function on their own. At the time, it seemed that there were just as many failures as successes, and the failures were colossal failures. One of the first Northampton patients I took care of was a woman who was admitted because she had burned herself in a suicide attempt. I worked with her for much of my four years there, until she was deinstitutionalized and transferred to a halfway house. She ended up burning herself alive along with several others. On the local news broadcast the announcer described a fire in an apartment in Holyoke, in which people were killed. I can still remember seeing the film of her body being carried out on a stretcher, covered with a blanket.

After four years at Northampton I was getting worn down myself and ready for a change. Because many of the doctors at the hospital didn't speak English very well, one of my jobs was to translate for them. I was pretty familiar with the psychotropic medications, and would suggest, "Maybe this patient should be put on that medicine." And frequently the doctors would take my advice. I began thinking to myself, "This guy is getting paid three or four times what I'm getting paid but I'm coming up with his prescriptions!"

In fact, I kept thinking I should have been a psychiatrist. When I mentioned that to Annette one day, she said, "Well, why couldn't you be?"

"Well, because I'd have to go to medical school," I replied. And she said, "So?" So I guess my decision ultimately to go to medical school was a little selfish because it was based on finances.

With Annette's encouragement I went back to school to take several science courses and then I took the Medical College Admission Test better known as the MCAT. We had saved $3000 to try to buy a house, but used the money on medical school applications—13 schools in all. Every single one rejected me! It was terrible.

But then I talked to my younger brother, who had gone about the process the old-fashioned way, applying right out of Holy Cross and getting accepted into Loyola School of Medicine, a Catholic school in Chicago. After I had gotten all my rejections, he called me up and told me, "Mark, you should apply to Loyola again for early decision. They tend to take the out-of-state people through the early decision program, then fill in the rest of the class with in-state people."

So I did, and I got lucky this time. For my admissions interview, I stayed at my brother's house in Chicago. He was on call, and his wife was at home with their three kids. The morning of my interview was crazy; we were all rushing around getting the kids dressed and fed. My sister-in-law dropped me off with one of the children at Loyola while she parked the car and tended to the other two. I remember running down the hall to my first interview carrying my two-year-old nephew. But somehow I managed to get to the interview on time and was accepted to study at Loyola.

Then I had to figure out a way to pay for med school. So I joined the Air Force—they paid the bills.

At age 30 I began my four years of med school at Loyola with the intention of becoming a psychiatrist. My first two years were all academic lecture classes, followed by two years of clerkships. We'd go through all the rotations—pediatrics, adult medicine, psychiatry, surgery—and as I progressed through them, I found them *all* very interesting. Meanwhile, Annette was observing all this and listening to my comments. Finally, she said to me, "Do you really want to go into psychiatry? Maybe you should think about family medicine. You like to do a little bit of everything, and in family practice you can even do a little bit of psychiatry." Well, that was true. You do end up doing a lot of garden-variety psychiatry in a primary care office. I was smart so I listened to my wife.

Because of my commitment to the Air Force, I did my residency in family medicine at Andrews Air Force Base, right outside of Washington, D.C. That lasted for three years, and after that, I owed the Air Force four years of service. They sent me to Wurtsmith Air Force Base in upstate Michigan. The mission of that base was to fly B-52s over the polar ice cap and bomb Russia—or not! The base was closed in 1993.

My family and I were in Michigan for a year and then went to Osan Air Force Base in Korea, about 40 miles south of Seoul. While we were living in Chicago, we had befriended a Korean family that lived downstairs from us. The husband was studying to be an orthodontist. Since they were now living in Seoul, we thought it would be cool to go to Korea and meet up with them, and that we did!

We had a fabulous time in Korea. We found that the country-side was very much like New England with rolling hills, although rice paddies replaced the dairy farms we were used to. The shopping was great—Annette liked that part. Plus, whenever we were on leave, we were able to travel in the Pacific. One year we spent Christmas in Hawaii. It cost us $10 each to fly to Hawaii, and then another $30 a day to stay in a little bungalow near the ocean.

Another time, we went on vacation to Alaska and I met up with Dave Harnisch, an old friend and running partner whom I knew when we were both residents at Andrews in Washington. At the time he was a physician at Eielson Air Force Base in Fairbanks. Dave really impressed me. It's kind of ironic that even though I was born Catholic, raised Catholic, went to Catholic high school, Catholic college and Catholic medical school, it wasn't until I got into the Air Force and met this truly devout Catholic doctor that I began to really understand what being a Catholic doctor meant.

That understanding centered on life issues, specifically contraception. I was a freshman at Holy Cross, a pretty liberal place in 1968 when *Humanae Vitae* was issued.[34] The response was unbelievable. "What's wrong with the Church? Why can't they get with it? They're so old and antiquated." Even the Jesuits at the college said, "Well, it just means that you should be open to having children at some point in your marriage." They weren't really supportive of what Pope Paul VI said, and so as I went through college, neither was I. Even though I kind of agreed with everything in *Humanae Vitae*, I remember feeling sort of disillusioned. But maybe "disillusioned" is too strong a word. Maybe it was more a feeling of embarrassment. Why can't the Church get with it? Why couldn't they moderate their position a bit? Why did they need to have such a hard line against contraception? When I got to Loyola, a Catholic medical school, there was no talk of *Humanae Vitae* or of natural family planning. All the Catholic doctors there prescribed birth control and so I did too. I figured that, in modern medicine, I had to do what the patients expected of me.

As Dr. Harnisch and I talked, we got on the topic of his work in the Couple to Couple League, where he taught the sympto-thermal method of natural family planning. I thought, "Hmm, that's kind of interesting." I wondered a little about why this person of science was doing something so "un-scientific." But I listened and later talked with Annette. We had four children by then and decided, "Why not have the Harnischs teach us this method of NFP?" So they did. Annette and I wished we had practiced NFP all along.

At that point I was still prescribing birth control but Dr. Harnish was not. For about a year I struggled with that but I rationalized the practice by thinking, "Just because I'm buying into this for myself doesn't mean I can push it on other people." But

34. *Humanae Vitae* (*Of Human Life*) was Pope Paul VI's encyclical on human sexuality, marriage and fertility published in 1968. The encyclical re-affirmed the traditional teaching of the Catholic Church regarding abortion and contraception and was controversial because of its prohibition of all forms of artificial contraception.

acting on one's Catholic faith isn't just for Catholics. We believe this is something that is natural law and should apply to all people. So when I left the Air Force and went into private practice, I decided it was a good time to make the break and I stopped prescribing contraceptives.

Coming back to Fitchburg was an easy decision. Both Annette and I had family there and we'd had our fill of traveling with the Air Force. Around this time I met another Catholic physician, Dr. Paul Carpentier, a family physician in the nearby town of Gardner.[35] He was approaching his medical practice from a similar point of view. Dr. Carpentier had studied the medical applications of NFP (known as NaProTech or Natural Procreative Technology) with Dr. Tom Hilgers at the Pope Paul VI Institute in Omaha. I was intrigued and so I took the course myself in the early 1990s and started using NaProTech in my medical practice. I then became trained to teach the method.

My evolving understanding of *Humanae Vitae* has really strengthened my faith. When I finally realized that everything Pope Paul VI said in that document came true—that increasingly available contraception would lead to more promiscuity, disrespect toward women, abortion, and broken families—it was a really life-changing, practice-changing concept for me. What I really came to see was that of all people, we doctors should be fostering a culture of life. It was depressing to see how far removed the medical profession was from that attitude; how it was signing on to the culture of death, with contraception, abortion, physician-assisted suicide, and artificial reproductive technologies. The basis of my own understanding hinged on *Humanae Vitae*.

Just last weekend I was asked by my pastor to speak to a confirmation class about Catholic sexual morality. I spent some time thinking about how to talk to the class and in doing that I reflected on my own medical practice. So many times, things come up that present a choice between the culture of life and the culture of death.

This choice has come up more than once for me. Here is one example of how it is called into play: I'm on call for another doctor, and I get a call from that doctor's patient, a young woman. She says, "I had unprotected sex last night and I need Plan B. Can you call in a prescription for me for the morning-after pill?" I say, "Well, gee, no. I can't do that."

---

35. Dr. Paul Carpentier is the subject of Chapter 4 of this book.

The patient says, "What? You can't do that? I'm the patient; you're the doctor. You've got to give me what I want."

I reply that Plan B is abortive. It's contraceptive in some respects, but it also causes early abortions. Then I tell the patient I don't believe in that.

Here's another example. Once a patient came to me asking for a vasectomy. He was married with three kids. I explained that I don't refer for those. At some point in our conversation he asked me, "Are you Catholic?" I told him that I am, and that as a Catholic, I don't believe in sterilization. But also, I said, I took an oath as a doctor to do no harm, and a vasectomy is doing harm because it is destroying a normal function, and a doctor should not do this. Fertility is not a disease, and contraception and sterilization are not health care. This particular patient was a faith-filled person from a Protestant denomination, and he was receptive to what I said. I explained that when you give yourself to your spouse in intercourse, you should be giving your whole self. If you say, "I give all of myself to you, but not my fertility," then you're *not* giving your whole self. And at some level it impairs your relationship.

Here is another example—and I can't tell you how many times this has happened. A young man comes in to see me. As I take the history I ask, "Are you married or single?" He replies, "Single."

"Do you have any children?" "Yes I have three children."

"Do you have any relationship with the mother of your children?" "Oh, yeah, we've been living together for years."

That's not something I'm going to jump on right away, but I will make a mental note of it. Here you have somebody who has, for all practical purposes, a wife and children who are dependent on him, and for all I know, he's acting like a good father. But if, in spite of that, he still considers himself single, how committed really is he? Certainly, whatever you say in those situations, you have to say in a caring way. You don't want to blow people off—you want instead to help them understand.

Since the 1960s, marriage in our society has become more and more meaningless, and this is related to the use of contraception, just as *Humanae Vitae* predicted. Contraception made cohabitation easier, and if you can have sex without babies, why not have two men or two women together? And then really, if you can have two men, why not three men, or three men and two women? Marriage becomes meaningless—pointless.

One of the things I brought up when I talked to the confirmation class was another situation that comes up in my practice. Sometimes when I am doing a physical on a teenager, I'll ask him if he's had any health education classes. If he says yes I'll ask him what he's been learning about. At some point he'll tell me that they've been talking about sexually-transmitted disease, so I'll ask, "How are you learning to avoid STDs?" Nine times out of ten, the kid will say, "Use protection."

So we'll talk about that a little. Then I'll ask if "protection" always works. The answer, of course, is no. Once I get to know the patient a bit, we'll talk about how he's really better off waiting until he's married for sex. I'll tell him that there's no condom for your heart. If you get prematurely intimate with someone and then you break up, then try a relationship with someone else and that doesn't work out either, eventually it breaks your heart. That's what kids are not being told at school.

We docs are very busy and there's always pressure to see more patients. But family practice has been a good choice for me. My wife was right; I don't like doing the same thing over and over. My youngest patient is about one month old and my oldest is 101. The variety of people I see in my practice is very gratifying—people of all different ages and with all different problems. It's life in its whole spectrum.

I'm glad I'm doing what I'm doing. It's a privilege being a physician, having people talk to you, sharing their troubles, and trusting you with their lives. It's kind of humbling too. Just being present to people at important times in their lives, going through illness or crisis with them, and helping them through transitions is really gratifying. Sure, the crazy hours and the paperwork can get to be hassles but even they don't overshadow the joy of the one-on-one with patients.

My practice of faith is a day-to-day thing. I try to start each day with a devotion. I've experimented with a lot of different things: reading from religious books and magazines, going online to daily devotional sites. I remember a priest once told me, "When you go in to see each patient, you should ask yourself, 'How can I serve today?'" So that is how I try to orient myself each morning.

My father used to start his day with a prayer called the Morning Offering. Each morning, he would say, "I offer You my prayers, works, joys and sufferings of this day." One of his patients was our parish priest, and one year at Christmas he gave my father a statue of Mary. The statue was displayed on our stairway, between the first and second floor. A card with the Morning Offering was displayed next to the statue. Being a busy surgeon, my father didn't have time for much else, so on his way down the stairs, he would say that prayer and then head off to the hospital. He set a good example for me.

It's been important to me to make sure that the Faith is passed on to my children. They're grown now, and I think, for the most part, that has happened. When I was growing up, I myself didn't buy into everything in the Faith but making sure my kids were grounded in their faith was probably more important to me than anything else. Annette and I did that by talking about issues with the children as they came up.

I still find myself thinking about things my father said to me and my siblings, referring to certain passages in Scripture. For example, we five boys were often fighting. One day we were fighting on the way to church, and my father yelled at us his paraphrase of that line from the Bible, "If you have a fight with your brother, don't come to the altar! Go and make amends before you come."[36]

I try to say some of the same things to my kids. When they talk about doubts such as: "Is there really a God?" I'll tell them about Pascal's Wager. The wager is this: If you live your life believing in an afterlife and you're wrong and you die, you won't know you were wrong. But if you live your life as a nonbeliever and you're wrong and you die, you *are* going to know it! That's a pretty practical approach. I tell my kids things like: You can live your life believing you're a speck of dust floating in the cosmos, or you can believe you're a child of God destined for immortality. How do you want to live *your* life? We've had hundreds of conversations like this as they were growing up.

Annette and I have been blessed with four children. Our oldest, Dorothy is married to a great guy and has four children and a stepchild. In addition to being a busy mom, she is an ICU nurse. We had a son, Timothy, who died in infancy. He was born with pulmonary stenosis, a heart defect. It was difficult for all of us, but it was especially difficult for Dorothy, his sister. She was only four when her brother was born and died. For a long time after that, her play consisted of building cemeteries.

---

36. "Therefore, if you bring your gift to the altar, and there recall that your brother has anything against you, leave your gift there at the altar, go first and be reconciled with your brother, and then come and offer your gift." (Mat 5:23-24)

That was an instructive time for us. Timothy was baptized shortly after birth. When we learned he had a heart defect, we were told he had to have a cardiac catheterization, during which he could possibly die. So we called up the medical school chaplain. The regular chaplain wasn't there; another priest was covering for him. We asked about having Last Rites for the baby, and this priest told us, "A baby doesn't need Last Rites. The baby doesn't have any sin. You don't have to worry about that."

The next day, the regular chaplain was back on duty. Fr. Lovely was his name, and he was a lovely man and priest, very soft-spoken. We asked again for Last Rites for our baby, and he said, "Oh, sure." He got us together and we performed the Last Rites but Timothy got through the catheterization. Later, when he was scheduled for surgery, we requested and received Last Rites for him again.

Timothy died during surgery, trying to repair the defect. He was a month old. We had his funeral in the hospital chapel. His body was in a little white casket. When we left the chapel, the only way we could roll the casket out was through the emergency department—any other way would have involved going down stairs. I remember the looks of all the people as we rolled out this tiny little casket.

My son's death didn't really make me doubt my faith. Bad things happen. Instead of saying, "Why me?" we can just as easily say, "Why not me?" It was a very difficult time, but it didn't make me think, "How could God do this to us?" Neither Annette nor I wanted to think that Timothy's death was the end. We wanted to think that we would see our son again someday. Faith makes that hope possible.

Timothy was buried in Queen of Heaven Cemetery outside of Chicago, in a special children's area. Near him are the graves of a group of babies who died in a tragic fire. And in that section of the cemetery is a statue of Jesus with the inscription: "Suffer the children to come unto Me, for thus is the Kingdom of God."[37] We took pictures of that statue. It was very consoling for us to think that our little one was going to God before us.

A year and a half after Timothy died, our son Quin was born. He's 26 now, and it's kind of funny, he's going down a path that's similar to mine. He earned his master's in mental health counseling and works with families of drug-addicted adolescents. Our "baby,"

---

37. Mat 19:14

Madeline, is 23. She was born in January, the same month as her brother Timothy, and Annette likes to say that she brought joy back to January for our family. She's working on a degree in physical therapy. All three of them are great kids and I think they're all growing up as good Catholic people.

I learned a lot about suffering from my son's illness and death. Several patients have also helped me see the redemptive quality of suffering. Suffering can be the result of bad choices, or it can stem from natural causes. Asking "Why did God let this happen?" never made sense to me, although I can understand it on an emotional level. But look what happened to Jesus Himself—He suffered mightily and died on a cross. How did His Father let that happen? Yet from suffering comes meaning and from suffering can come redemption.

I think of one patient in particular: a woman, whose younger brother has cerebral palsy and suffered severe brain damage at birth. He's now 40 years old; she's about five years older. She has her own children but he is like another child. He's totally uncommunicative. The only sounds he can make are grunts. She takes him to appointments and all the places he needs to go. You could say, "Why did that have to happen to this guy?" But I think that, in a very real sense, her brother is a vehicle for her salvation. She's a better person because of him. If you look at suffering like that, I think it strengthens your faith rather than makes you lose it.

I know a young guy in his 30s, Billy, who is a caretaker for a brain-damaged cerebral palsy patient who's around 50 and is totally nonverbal. The patient, Jim, carries a radio around and spends half his time banging himself on the head. Yet Billy takes him everywhere. You can tell Billy cares for Jim because he wants every problem addressed and makes sure Jim gets everything he needs. Billy even takes Jim on vacation and buys him gifts. There's no familial relationship between them. Billy gets paid by the state for taking care of Jim, but he's certainly not paid enough. You have to really want to do that; you have to treat it as a vocation.

I asked Billy once, "Why do you do this?" He seemed confused. "What do you mean, why?" he said.

"How can you do what you do, caring so well for someone who is so severely impaired?"

He acted as if I were an idiot for asking him that. "Oh," he said, "It's very fulfilling, very gratifying."

In many ways Billy is sacrificing his own life by devoting himself to Jim's care. How much of a life can you have if you've always got this severely impaired person with you? But clearly, it's a good life for him. Cases like that teach me a lot. It's hard to pity myself when I see someone making that kind of sacrifice.

Annette and I are parishioners at St. Anthony of Padua in Fitchburg. I went there as a kid, was an altar boy, made my First Communion and my Confirmation, and got married there. Our children attended the parish's parochial school. We originally sent our children to a public elementary school. And then one day my son, who was in third grade at the time, came home and told us how he was learning about protected sex. When I went to talk to the principal about it, he was kind of apologetic but acted like he didn't know what was going on. Apparently the teacher was "free-lancing"—the discussion of protected sex was not part of the official third grade curriculum. They had been talking about HIV and about Ryan White, the hemophiliac boy who contracted AIDS through a blood transfusion. I have no idea how the teacher made the leap from Ryan White to protected sex. Annette and I decided, "That's it. We're outta here."

Not only did the children attend St. Anthony School, but I have served on the school's board of directors and Annette is an early childhood teacher at St. Anthony. She teaches three- and four-year-olds. I don't know how she does it. She comes home tired, but she loves it. She says, "I get to go to school and play every day!" The school is a big part of our life.

I used to teach high school level CCD myself on a regular basis, when I had more time. Now I just give occasional talks such as my recent one to the confirmation class. But I do find time to be a Eucharistic minister. I started doing that when we moved back to Massachusetts after the Air Force. I find so much meaning in that ministry. The priest explained to us that when you hold the Host in your hand and look at the other person and say "The Body of Christ," you're not just saying, "Here is the Body of Christ." You're saying, "You are the Body of Christ. I am the Body of Christ. We are the Body of Christ."

I think of what the priest told us when I serve as a Eucharistic minister. It's such an awesome thing to be holding the Creator of the universe in your hands. You can look at it in two ways. You can feel such awe and reverence that you don't even want to touch the Eucharist. But on the other hand, Christ came into the world as a vulnerable little baby. And you've *gotta* touch a baby! I like both those aspects of the Eucharist.

Early in the morning I attend weekly Eucharistic adoration at a perpetual adoration chapel in one of the local churches. They started it up about 10 years ago and were asking people to volunteer for one hour a week. I enjoy it, because otherwise I wouldn't take the time to sit and meditate for more than five minutes. During that hour, I'm usually alone. So I can really pray and sit in the presence of Jesus in the Blessed Sacrament. Being there also allows me to read something more substantial than a two-minute devotion. I admit that sometimes I find myself sleeping through it—then I feel guilty!

Eucharistic adoration is part of my weekly routine. Maybe it's the Catholic in me, but I just love rituals. Every Friday I like to go home after work and cook myself a couple of hot dogs. I'll watch the Red Sox or the Celtics and eat my hot dogs and beans, and that's how I know it's Friday. On Tuesdays I go to adoration, and we go to Church together on Sundays. It all gives life a rhythm.

Speaking of the Red Sox—I'm a huge fan. My office is something of a Red Sox "shrine." The walls are covered with memorabilia, including baseball cards, a vintage photo of Ted Williams at his first at-bat in a Red Sox uniform, and a panoramic shot of Fenway Park during the ceremony when the team received their 2004 World Series rings. I can show you where my family and I were in the stands that day. I even have a stuffed toy of the team mascot, Wally the Green Monster, for my young patients. When you press his hand, he dances and plays "Sweet Caroline," the Sox' eighth inning stretch song.

But my pride and joy is a photo of me holding the Red Sox 2004 World Series trophy. That photo was the product of an "epic" quest on my part. The trophy was being displayed for the fans in different Massachusetts towns, and I found out it was coming to a high school near Fitchburg. So I set out that day to see it. But I got lost and ended up running late. When I finally pulled in, the fans were all gone and the crew was packing the trophy into a van to take it away. I begged them to take it out for me and reluctantly, they did. "Could I please hold it?" I begged them. "No," they said, "We don't allow anybody to hold it."

"Well then," I pleaded, "could you please at least hold it next to me so I can get a picture of me *looking* like I'm holding it?" They rolled their eyes, but finally gave in and said, "Here. You can hold it."

One of the nice things about practicing here in Fitchburg is that my father was also the physician for many of my patients. In fact, when I first began practice here, my father and I were on the same hospital staff. Many of my older patients will tell me, "Oh, I knew your father. He took out my appendix," or "Your father saved my little girl." It's nice to hear these stories.

A nurse once told me that, years ago, she had been having abdominal pain and nobody could figure out what was wrong. She suffered a huge weight loss and really thought she was going to die. She finally went to my father and he said, "Well, let's do an exploratory." Think about what it was like being a surgeon in the days before ultrasounds and CAT scans—you had nothing to go on, you just went in. The old-time surgeons used to say, "Never let the abdominal wall stand between you and a diagnosis!" So my father operated on her and fixed her. I think the problem was a chronic abscess. She's been fine ever since. "Your father saved my life," she told me.

My father didn't usually give me overt advice. He was never the type to pick up the phone every week to say, "Mark, you should do this or that," except he *did* tell me, "You've got to go to Holy Cross!" But I would often call him; he was a great sounding board.

I am very fortunate to have had two loving and devout Catholic parents. I've spoken about my dad quite a bit, but I should also say that my mom has had a great impact on my life. She is passionately pro-life not only because she had six kids of her own but because she has also been a constant supporter of pro-life causes. After the infamous *Roe v. Wade* decision in 1973, she helped establish a local chapter of Massachusetts Citizens for Life as well as a local crisis-pregnancy center. At 88 years of age she is still engaged in life and going strong.

This month is the 13th anniversary of my father's death. My dad was healthy for most of his life. He was a very stoic guy and never complained. If he had problems, he just sucked it up. That's what most of his generation did. But when he was about 65 years old, he injured his shoulder. And even though it got badly infected, he wouldn't see a doctor. It's true what they say: Doctors make terrible patients. Finally, Annette, my wife, noticed that my father was wincing in pain when one of our children touched his shoulder.

She told me emphatically, "Your dad needs to see a doctor!" I put him in the car and took him in.

My dad was hospitalized immediately. He had staph sepsis and was on IV antibiotics for six weeks. He never really recovered from the infection. It wasn't long afterward that that he was diagnosed with Parkinson's disease. And when a surgeon gets Parkinson's... well, forget about surgery. My father said he would never retire. He used to say, "Retirement is something to contemplate but never to undertake." But in this case, he had no choice.

He was only 73 when he died. He and my mother used to go to Eucharistic adoration once a week. He was sitting in his favorite chair at home and my mother came in to tell him, "Well, it's time to leave for adoration." She left the room but didn't hear him get up or anything. When she went back in, he was dead. She called the paramedics, but there was nothing they could do. He probably died of an arrhythmia.

As I go about my work each day, I often think about my dad, particularly if I find references to him when I'm looking through old medical records on my patients. He set a good example for me.

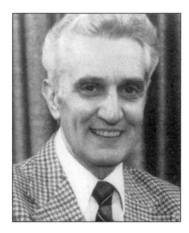

Dr. Quintino Rollo

— *Ad Majorem Dei Gloriam* —

10

Dr. Scot Bateman

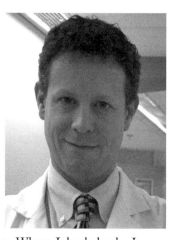

THE PIETA IN
THE PICU

The reasons why I went into the specialty of pediatric critical care and why I became a Catholic are very much tied together. Yet the rational side of me is completely at a loss to explain either one. When I look back, I realize that all the decisions I made along the way were guided by something I didn't understand. Both decisions involved a kind of brush with the divine and as with all major decisions in life, knowing that helps me retain a sense of wonder.

Growing up in Lake Tahoe, California, I wasn't completely without any spirituality, but it mostly centered around nature and the mountains. My mom grew up as a Christian Scientist; my dad considers himself Lutheran. We went to church perhaps five times during my whole childhood, but I knew the main stories: the Christmas pageant, the rock rolled away from the tomb. My father was a high school history teacher but after he and my mother divorced, when I was young, he became a family practice doctor. He had not wanted to be a doctor when he was growing up, but I certainly did. As a child, I would rush to a fallen friend on the playground and tell him that I could help because I was going to be a doctor some day. Somehow, it always seemed to work.

Despite that early inner pull, I went through Dartmouth College trying very hard *not* to become a doctor in large part because my father was discouraging me from pursuing a career in medicine. I was getting a strong liberal arts education and it seemed like there were so many available career paths. But after much deliberation, I found myself taking my first job as a lab technician studying inflammatory responses. One day someone at the lab questioned why I hadn't applied to med school. The very next day, I did just that because I couldn't understand myself why I hadn't applied all those years ago. I entered Dartmouth Medical School with much excitement and far more focus than I had in college, because I felt I was allowing myself to be true to what I was destined to be. My faith journey at this point was more about following my calling as a physician than about any kind of overt religious response. I was listening, learning to appreciate and allowing that calling to guide me in big decisions.

I earned my medical degree, and then went on to Children's Hospital in Boston for my residency and fellowship. I had originally put pediatrics last on my list of intended specialties in medical school. I had already decided to go into internal medicine and had even filled out the paperwork. Pediatrics was not something that interested me. I felt that it was mostly a lot of well-child check-ups and involved less physiology and less learning about diseases. But when I did it in my last rotation, I was shocked to realize that I really did want to specialize in pediatrics. My wife, whom I had married during medical school, was also very surprised. I found that the physiology and the need to apply medicine are definitely important and that there is also an intrinsic humanism and a need to work closely with the family unit. Because I believed this was the way medicine should be practiced, I knew pediatrics was the right calling for me and it was what I needed to do.

At the start of my first rotation as a pediatric intern in the ICU at Children's Hospital, like most residents, I was remarkably naïve and had so much to learn. But the many patients who came through that environment stayed with me. I can recall my first patient, Hayley, who died there. She was born prematurely and suffered from chronic lung disease, complicated by an RSV infection that just ravaged her lungs and despite our best efforts, her condition deteriorated. Some time after her death, I received a card from her mom, telling me how grateful she was for my care of Hayley and how much I had helped her despite her death. I was astonished to learn that even though the little girl had died, in some small way I had made a difference in the life of this child.

Another one of my patients, an 11-year-old girl named Emily, taught me something about the nature of grace. She suffered from acute lymphoblastic lymphoma but despite chemotherapy she was found to have more metastases. When the time came to give her the news of her prognosis, she asked me— curiously, earnestly, fearfully—"Scot, what's it going to feel like when I die?"

The question brought me up short. Nobody had taught me how to answer that in med school. But her look demanded honesty. After a long pause thinking about the unknown and the unknowable, and hoping that the words came out right, I said slowly, "It will probably feel like you're falling deeper and deeper asleep. You'll find it harder and harder to wake up and see us all here. And finally you won't be able to wake up at all. Instead you'll be in your dreams from then on." There was a silence as she absorbed this. Then she looked at me directly and said, "I like my dreams."

We both shed tears of sorrow, but in her relief, release, and acceptance, I was able to see, for the first time, grace, pure and simple. She died a week later, but I have to believe that her death was a peaceful one.

There were victories during this phase of my career as well. When I was an intern, I took care of a newborn named Scott, who spent three weeks on a heart-lung bypass machine. My care of him involved providing the highly technical support needed for this machine, but also being there for his family during his long weeks of treatment. The treatment worked and he did great. By now, I assume he would be about 14 years old.

I was once told that if you can talk yourself out of working in the ICU, you should do it. But I couldn't, nor could my wife. The conventional wisdom is that it doesn't make sense to want to be around trauma, pain and suffering all the time and that given the choice, most people would run away from them as fast as they could. But the people who work in the ICU seem to be there for the right reasons—not for money or glory or prestige. These people have a desire to be present to help families in pain. Seeing them give of themselves and sensing their faith in each other was very enlightening to me. My decision to stay in the PICU didn't make rational sense at the time. Rather, it was almost a form of surrender to something that allowed me to be true to myself. I felt what I was doing was meaningful and I wanted to learn as much as I could. Was it a decision based on faith? I would not have called it that at the time, but looking back now I would say, yes, it was faith that guided me.

I have found that you cannot be around suffering too long before you want to try to understand it. You can't see an innocent child on a ventilator, severely injured or sick, and not question why they are suffering. But then you need to be able to function and not be buried by the intensity of the situation. A sick child really tugs at everyone's heartstrings. To witness families searching for comfort, help, and stability puts their suffering right in your face. These searches are universal, whether the family is Muslim, Protestant, Catholic, voodoo practitioners, or agnostic. What they need at these times is a sense of God and of the divine. Their longing resonated in me, because it meshed with my own sense of spirituality.

I was in the process of absorbing these insights when a question from Ann, a Catholic physician and colleague of mine, took me by surprise. We were discussing a patient who had died when she asked me, "Where is God in your life?" I paused a long time because I really had no meaningful answer for that question. I finally responded lamely that I felt closest to God when I was in the mountains. But that wasn't really a satisfactory answer because it was pretty evident that I didn't spend a lot of time in the mountains.

Ann's question, and my lack of a sound answer, made it clear that deep inside me was some sense of faith, trust and belief, even though I had no substantial religious background. I could not name these feelings; I had no vocabulary with which to have a conversation about them. I was completely unable to articulate what I had felt inside of me. But I recognized that some guiding force had been calling me throughout my life and my practice and had played a major role in my decisions. My inability to provide a coherent answer left me at a loss and looking for a way to better explain things. I guess the Holy Spirit was finally saying, "I have been right here, just get to know Me better."

And so my official faith journey began after this conversation with Ann. I became more directed toward the Catholic Church, because that was where I felt a connection with the sacredness that I also connected with in the PICU. I began reading, thinking, and learning about what Jesus taught, about why Catholic means "universal," and about what these concepts meant for me. As I read, I found myself saying, "Yes, of course, that makes sense, that's what I felt." It wasn't as if I was discovering something new as much as I was confirming and validating my own experience in a very lovely way. I had found a friend to be with me and give me guidance.

This awakening of my faith was closely tied to an atmosphere of discord that was building between my wife and me. Most of it was related to the stresses of being a committed physician who wasn't home enough, but faith issues also became a source of conflict in my marriage. My wife was fine with my exploration of different religions as long as it was not Catholicism. This bias stemmed from a childhood experience in which her babysitter kept trying to convert her and her family to the Catholic faith. As a result, she viewed the Catholic Church as very negative and rigid. I thus tried very hard to find some other faith outlet and while my "church-shopping" confirmed for me that all the faiths were looking for the same thing, I still found myself sneaking off to the Catholic Church for Mass. I wanted the sacredness of the Eucharist and I couldn't find that anywhere else. This awareness drove my sense that the Catholic Church was where I needed to be.

Then, in 2002, I found myself in Atlanta for a physicians' conference, and on a Sunday morning I walked into Sacred Heart Church, not far from the hotel where I was staying. It was Pentecost Sunday. I had no idea what "Pentecost" meant. But as the celebration of the Mass continued, I found myself drawn to receive Communion. I knew I wasn't supposed to do this, but the call was irresistible.

So I ate the Body, and drank the Blood, and when I went back to my pew, an indescribable sense of warmth flowed through me. It began in the pit of my stomach and spread to my limbs, to the pews, to the people around me, to the stained glass windows, to the bricks, to the mortar. I was in communion with everything around me. I began to weep uncontrollably because of an intense combination of unworthiness and awe at the existence of God and love. When I stopped crying, the church was empty and the Mass was over. Then I began to laugh just as uncontrollably as I had wept, knowing that nobody would ever believe what had just happened to me. I felt a profound sense of sadness because of all that I had not known for all of those years, as well as a sense of joy for the beauty, the feeling of peace, and the understanding of Truth that had come over me.

So now that I'd had this experience, the question became what was I going to do about it. My wife and I were going through a very difficult time. We had even started marriage counseling. Yet I could not understand how I could be feeling such a close connection to God and the Church and at the same time be viewed so negatively in my own home. We were all going through hell, including our two children who were just two and four years old at the time. I felt like the blind man from the wonderful Gospel story, who was touched by Christ and then able to see. But also in that story, his neighbors turned against him and claimed they didn't know him. Even his own parents wouldn't support him. Despite my new vision, I too, was feeling that kind of rejection.

Finally, I hit bottom. We had been going through a particularly bad time. One day, I was literally lying on my office floor, turning all these things over in my mind and trying to figure out what to do. I finally was moved to get up off the floor and I went straight to St. Ignatius Church. Sitting there in the pew, I agonized over how this journey to God could be so painful and yet so beautiful. Finally, I decided that I couldn't rationalize anymore. I closed my eyes and said out loud "Well, God, it's in your hands. I'm done."

At that moment, the organ started playing, which shook me up a bit. When I opened my eyes, there in front of me stood Tony, one of my preceptors from Children's Hospital. After Mass was over, I decided to share with him my interest in the Church. He introduced me to the director of religious education, who told me about the parish's Open Arms program, which helped people understand Catholicism.

The next night, I went to my first Open Arms meeting and told them I didn't know why I was there, but that I had plenty of questions. A lot of them were superficial: Why do we stand for the Gospel but not for the Old Testament readings? Why is this sacrament more important than something else? "You need to explain this to me," I kept saying. "We've got a live one here!" joked Father Bob, who presided over the Open Arms program. After 10 weeks of asking every question under the sun, I entered the Rite of Christian Initiation for Adults. I became very close to Father Bob and the people in RCIA at St. Ignatius and met with them many times outside of church-related functions. Tony ended up being my sponsor and godfather at my initiation into the Church at the Easter Vigil in 2004. After I had gone through the waters of baptism, I felt fresh and alive, with an incredible sense of familiarity, as if I was home again. I haven't missed a Sunday Mass since my baptism—going there is something I look forward to doing.

People who are cradle Catholics may not appreciate what it's like not to have access to the Eucharist. My experience of not having it, then having it and then not having it again (during the RCIA process) underscored for me the connection it provides. It manifests an ongoing, intimate relationship with God that's beautiful, nourishing, and induces such gratitude.

Being without the Eucharist left me filled with longing.

I found that I was especially drawn to the insistence on the sacredness of the Eucharist in the Catholic Church. I believe that if you have something that's sacred, you should treat it that way. If you had a magic wand that your ancestors had kept for 2000 years and that could be used to change things, you would treat it as sacred. That wand would be kept in a special box and treated with infinite care and you'd want to pass it on. That's what you'd expect someone to do with something they considered as important as God. The Church's insistence that the Eucharist be treated with the utmost respect really resonated with me. I had experienced this same sense of the sacred in the PICU, where we treated patients and families with the utmost respect.

However my involvement with RCIA was the final dagger, the final symbol of betrayal, to my wife. We split up and I lived in a small one-bedroom apartment nearby. This eventually led to her filing for divorce. I was alone and broken from the divorce. This was the darkest time of my life, what I call my hermit phase, which lasted a couple of years. But it was also a time of incredible spiritual growth, deflating my pride, leading me to spend a great deal of time in prayer and reading poetry. I slowly emerged out of the darkness and was given a fresh start.

My former colleague Ann (the one who had asked me where God was in my life) had been in Philadelphia during my divorce and my conversion to Catholicism. After I was baptized, I called her up and said, "Hey, let's talk about this again." This led to further spiritual discussions, and then eventually led to another question, "Are you still single?" We conversed long distance for a while, then began dating. Going to Mass with her was a new experience for me. Sharing a faith and keeping God in the center was so beautiful. We eventually grew closer and closer and decided to get married in the Church. Since neither my ex-wife nor I had been baptized when we were married we were granted the Petrine Privilege, in which a non-sacramental, or natural, marriage is dissolved by the Holy See, with the Pope as the final adjudicator. The process is fairly uncommon and it took a year to go through Rome. That was quite painful in its own way; here I was, a new member of the Church, and yet I was exposed to all of the church's inner workings as well as the bureaucracy and its lack of appreciation for how difficult this is for the former spouses. And of course my ex-wife wasn't happy about it either.

These days I have a good relationship with my ex-wife. We have two children that we share and they always come first. I go with her to parent-teacher nights at the kids' school and since she too has remarried, our kids now have four parents on the sidelines for sporting events. On the days I am not with them, I speak with my children on the phone. It still hurts not to be with them daily, but I have to believe that my faith has helped me to be a better father to them and their lives are now peaceful.

My kids, who are now 10 and 12, are with me every other weekend and they come to Mass with Ann and me. Their faith life is still something of an area of contention; they've been officially blessed in the Unitarian Church, which isn't recognized as baptism in the Catholic Church. I go back and forth between feeling that I should be more insistent on their early Catholic upbringing versus allowing them to be led by the Holy Spirit as they mature. I'm counting on my own practice of faith to guide my children as they form their own relationships with God. Going to church is not something we can argue about, we just go. That's what we do. Their religious upbringing is a complicated situation, but I'm hopeful that my own witness to faith is moving them. They are getting more curious, which is nice, and I tell them, "If you want to know more about it, just let me know." My wife, Ann, is great at explaining things too, and they see our connection to each other and to our faith. I guess we'll see how the Holy Spirit moves them as time goes on.

I've realized in my work with families in the PICU that whoever we are, we're all searching for the same things: faith, hope, and love. How we get there is a very individual journey and very much based on our own culture. Everyone needs to find their own path in their own best possible way. Every religion has its little quirks, but they all have the same goal, the same desire, the same force driving them. This universality gives me as a Catholic physician the ability to relate to and to appreciate the power of all religious faiths.

I see people's faith through our shared experiences in the PICU, and work with them, one family at a time, as they deal with their tragedies. To be able to help them, to comfort them, to give them trust and hope is really all I can do. I see in the PICU all the concepts taught in the Bible—suffering, hope, faith, rebirth—and they are more powerful than anything I can say.

Early in my conversion process, I saw an image of Michelangelo's *Pieta* for the first time. This work of art really struck a chord in me. I could completely understand this image of a mother caring for her dying Son, because I found I was seeing this over and over again in the PICU. I saw parents lying on the bed next to their child, hands clasped in prayer. I saw mothers whose faces were full of pain and woe, tenderly cradling their infants as they breathed their last.

The Crucifix also became alive to me in the PICU. For example, a little 10-year-old boy had an innocent accident that left him with a severe head injury and in need of mechanical ventilation. His arms were outstretched and lines were running into his veins; his brains were all wrapped up. It was uncanny how much his position resembled Jesus on the Cross. I've begun to see love when I see the Crucifix and to appreciate that love can happen even in the face of tragedy such as Jesus being crucified. To know, that despite the suffering, love is still present—to see that in the outpouring of love from families to their kids—is a privilege for me.

People ask, "How can you deal with all that suffering every day?" It's true that we see people at their worst, but their behavior is coming from a place of love. Parents get frightened when their child is in danger. Because they love that child far beyond any comprehension, their fears intensify. Yet at the same time they can be at their best. The love and the sustenance they provide to their children—that side of humanity—is truly beautiful to see. To appreciate that helps me deal with anxious parents.

Part of my job is to help my staff and the residents who come to our unit see that beauty in the face of suffering, to appreciate human dignity, and to cultivate respect for all of our patients. When the new residents come in every month, they're seeing all this for the first time. Helping them navigate the emotional minefield they're experiencing here is very enlightening for me. I'm one of the adherents of Saint Francis of Assisi—he is said to have taught, "Preach the gospel at all times, and when necessary, use words." I try to be a witness in the way we approach the care of our patients by dealing with them one patient at a time.

I have found some other resources helpful in my spiritual growth. The Spiritual Exercises of St. Ignatius were a wonderful format for learning different types of prayer—centering prayer, guided imagery prayer—for different situations. I was also touched by the Joshua books by Father Joseph Girzone, which I studied at the right time before my conversion really began. The *Joshua* books convey who Jesus is as a person in a lovely simple way. They are a beautiful, simple expression of faith. I've also become fond of the writings of Thomas Merton, particularly *No Man is an Island*. I love his writing. He has a way of explaining simplicity—the humility of "letting go and letting God"—that resonates with me. I also appreciate the fact that, like me, he was a convert to the Faith. I love reading conversion stories, like the story of St. Paul; they are a testament to the power and the mystery of God. I took Luke as my confirmation name because like me, he was a physician and a convert.

I'm very lucky that my wife Ann's faith is extremely important to her. She too is a physician and her practice of medicine is very faith-based. It's really enriching for us to discuss how we approach medicine. The way she cares for and interacts with her patients is beautiful to see.

I definitely treat the PICU as a sacred place. We don't do anything ritualistic there, but I still go around there in a prayerful state. I believe that taking care of patients and being of service is a form of prayer. I have a copy of *The Physician's Prayer* on the wall of my office and I pray it when I've had a bad day or when I know it's going to be a bad day. Part of the prayer asks God to take away anything that might interfere with my being of service and trying to best utilize my skills and other qualities. The prayer reminds me that I'm just trying to be a good servant.

Because my job in the ICU is totally focused on helping people deal with tragedy, I don't let myself get buried by asking why God would allow tragedy to happen. Is it totally unfair? Yes. Why does it happen? I can't explain that. It's as impossible to answer that question as it is to explain why the World Trade Center towers were attacked on September 11, 2001. As soon as you get involved in asking "why," it becomes hard to deal with a true theological perspective that's helpful.

I like to say that it's not what happens that is important, but how we deal with it. How we deal with it has a lot to do with God. Things happen that are beyond our control, but when patients get here, we do everything we can to help them and their parents get through their tragedy. My staff feels very much the same. While patients are here, they deserve the best, and that's what we strive to give them.

I recently finished a five-month course in clinical pastoral education for health care providers. The course involved a lot of sharing and introspection about experiences and conversations we've had with patients on spiritual topics. It was eye-opening, and definitely worthwhile for me to take. When I was in med school, there was little or no acknowledgement of patients' spiritual needs. But recently, I think medical schools have tried to include more of this type of education in their training.

The course in clinical pastoral education gave me a language and a structure that allows me to tell patients and families that we're open to their spiritual needs, that we think those needs are important and that we are willing to help. These types of conversations are different for every family, because every family is in a different place. I could ask formalized questions about religious practices or experiences, but I prefer to probe gently and see where the conversation goes.

These conversations typically start with an acknowledgement of the family's stress and pain. We talk about the patient's pain all the time, but at some point I try to redirect the dialogue to determine what the family is going through. The question can be as simple as "Did you get any sleep last night?" which often provides me with an insight into what their experiences are like. Often they feel helpless and scared because they don't have any control over their kid. By letting them know that "Yes, I care about what you're experiencing too," I find that faith emerges in our dialogues. When a person is out of control, scared and helpless, more often than not, faith is the next thing on his or her agenda; it's right there at the surface. The ensuing conversation might not be a deep theological discussion. It may be as simple as me saying, "I'm off duty this weekend and I'll be praying for you." And if a family member tells me that they have been praying a lot for the child, I say, "That is as important as anything medical we can offer. We'll take all the help we can get."

I've had to deal with a lot of questions about why I became a Catholic from my family and friends, who view the Church as a system of rules and dogma. To complicate matters, the clergy sexual abuse scandal was at its height at the time I converted. But for me, taking the Eucharist is a relationship that the Holy Spirit allows you to have with God through your faith. It also allows you to appreciate that God is not trying to dictate to you from above but rather is trying to guide you from below. The Church's teachings are supposed to be leading us into a deeper relationship with God. That's why it's important to hear the Pope speaking to us, trying to infuse us with his thoughts and beliefs so that we can integrate them into our daily lives.

For me, one of the basic aspects of faith is to live a life of simplicity. By that I mean being able to live day by day, to "love one another as I have loved you."[38] Our culture is trying to make everything so complex. Jesus didn't leave too many instructions. His message was very simple: We should get back to treating others the way we would want to be treated. To my joy, my daughter, the older of the two, has also adopted that sense of simplicity and my son is getting there.

My work in the PICU can certainly be complex. There's so much high technology at our disposal, and my responsibility as a doctor is to know what's available and what's the best for each child, because I believe that every child deserves the best. That's the simplicity of it. Sure, there are nuances—that's part of doing what's best for each patient. Do I get bogged down with policies and procedures? Definitely. Sometimes policies take away from the individuality of each patient. But when we focus on being present for the families who need us, we receive a reward that is more meaningful than anything we can imagine and that is a deepest of thanks.

There are times when we've given our best but, in spite of that, patients die. Sometimes we find that we have to help people change what they're hoping for. I often tell families that we can hope for the best, but we must prepare for the worst, and sometimes that means hoping for a sense of dignity at the end of life. Solid research tells us that a family's ability to cope with a child's death is related to their belief in the transcendence of the parent-child relationship. If we know a child's survival is out of the question, then we can hope that we can help a family come to terms with its loss. This realization is something that I did not appreciate early in my career.

Once I had a family come up to me in the hospital and thank me for what I had done for their son. I wracked my brain but could not remember who they were. I found out later that they had been in the ICU with their son for just four hours before he died and that I had walked out of there thinking I was a failure because I had lost the child. However, their appreciation for my help made me see failure in a new way. It goes far beyond what I can do with medicine or an IV. It's far greater than that and that's what I try to hold onto.

When I look back on my life I see it has been full of mysteries such as how I came to the PICU, how I came to faith.

38. John 13:34

I realize that all of the decisions I have made along the way were guided by something I didn't understand at the time. I feel, though, that somehow my life has been guided by something divine. Knowing that gives me a deep sense of gratitude and awe.

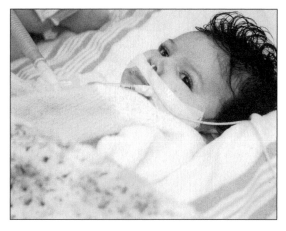

Isabella, born with Spinal Muscular Atrophy,
lovingly pictured in the PICU shortly
before her death.

— *Ad Majorem Dei Gloriam* —

11

Rebecca Ackroyd
Second-year medical student

WIPING CHRIST'S TEARS

When I was in high school, I liked just about every available career choice. I wanted to be everything—an astronaut, a teacher, a missionary, a firefighter, a doctor. My mother was the one who pointed out, "If you were a doctor, you could do several of those things. You could help people, you could travel, you could do mission work, you could teach." I thought about what she said and I decided to become a doctor. Although there have been moments of doubt since then, I am now a second-year medical student at the University of Massachusetts.

After graduating from high school, I went to college at Notre Dame and majored pre-med. But when I came home for Christmas in my freshman year, everything was up in the air. One evening in the kitchen, I had a conversation with my parents. I told them I wasn't sure if I was in the right major, if medicine was it for me. I was in some science classes I really didn't enjoy, and I thought that if pre-med was this miserable, then I didn't want to go to medical school.

But I was encouraged by several doctors I know. When I talked to them about it, they told me that a lot depends on the med school you attend. Some schools, they told me, are very competitive but some are not. I knew that I didn't like a competitive atmosphere.

The decision to continue in medicine really solidified for me during the summer after my junior year, when I got a grant from Notre Dame for a two-month internship working in a medical clinic in the mountains of the Dominican Republic. I went into that summer praying, "God, I really want to be a doctor but I don't want to go to med school and I kind of have to do the one to be the other. Help me see if med school is going to be worth it." That internship proved to be my dream job. I loved it, absolutely loved it. I came home determined that working in clinics in developing countries was the kind of work I wanted to do.

I was one of two students from Notre Dame who worked at the clinic that summer. The doctors treated both of us like med students, even though we were just college students. They taught us to suture patients, to give shots, to dress wounds, to put in IVs. I thought it was *so* cool. I loved it so much that sometimes I would lie to my friends who wanted me to come to town with them for a swim. I'd tell them I had to work, but really I didn't. All I wanted to do was to be at the hospital.

The town I worked in was a rural community of 20,000 people high in the mountains. But the geographic area of the town was small, the houses were closely packed together, and there were a lot of people living in each house. People didn't have a lot of personal space as we do here.

My understanding of poverty fundamentally changed with that experience. I made a friend in the town and remember going to her house to share a dinner that she cooked. I discovered that she had to borrow an extra bowl and spoon from a neighbor for me. She had nothing in her house except two chairs, a bed and a camp stove. Before working in the Dominican Republic, I totally would have called that poverty. But at the time, I thought, "She's not poor. We're borrowing a plate, but she has food. People down the street don't even have food." I also knew there were homeless people in the town, like the man who built a little shack on the sidewalk next to the hospital and used the hospital's bathroom. He often had nothing to eat. My time in the Dominican Republic made me re-evaluate what it means to have and to have not.

One incident during my work at the clinic raised an unexpected moral dilemma and taught me to be more careful before taking on a job. I was asked to assist in surgery, as one of the "pass-the-scalpel" people. I thought we were doing a C-section. When I scrubbed in, the patient was already out cold from the anesthesia and everyone was getting ready for the surgery. But as the procedure got underway, I realized that there was no baby in this woman's uterus and this was not a C-section. I thought, "Oh my gosh, what if this is a sterilization procedure? I shouldn't be assisting with this." I knew it was very common in that town, as well as throughout the country, for women to be surgically sterilized. I stood there, looking calm and normal on the outside, but my mind was racing a mile a minute.

Then the doctor handed me the woman's uterus and told me to put it in the trash can. That's when I realized that this poor woman was a cancer patient, not a patient undergoing sterilization. Obviously I felt compassion for her, but I also felt a huge sense of relief for myself. I decided that from then on, I would be sure to read the surgical schedule carefully.

The first time I actually saw someone die was at this hospital in the Dominican Republic. It happened on a night that I wasn't even scheduled to work. The patient, who was in her 30s, was mentally retarded. She was lying in a bed in the emergency room, waiting with her mother for the staff to decide whether or not to admit her. We were in and out attending to different patients. All of a sudden I heard someone sobbing and yelling very loudly. I turned around and saw that it was the mother, crying and almost screaming at her daughter who lay lifeless on the bed.

The doctors called for an oxygen tank, but no one seemed to be rushing and the oxygen took forever to arrive. I'm not sure if the woman was already dead and they were just going through the motions of trying to revive her for her mother's sake, or if she was still alive and they were only halfheartedly trying to revive her. Not having any medical training I didn't really understand what was happening. All I knew was what I could see—a young woman lying lifeless on the stretcher and her mother in great distress, sobbing. The staff tried to give her oxygen for a little while, then stopped, listened to the heart, and hearing nothing, declared the woman dead.

At that point my emotions kicked in and I felt so overwhelmed. I told the staff that I had to go home and I just took off. When I got home, I talked to my roommate a long time about what had happened, about life, death and other big issues. But although witnessing that death was pretty traumatic, it did not scare me away from medicine.

My undergraduate years at Notre Dame really helped to nurture my faith. When my parents met, my mother was Catholic and my father was Baptist, so when they married, they compromised and we attended Episcopal services. Eventually, after a new priest arrived whom my mother didn't like, she went back to the Catholic Church. From that point on, we split our Sundays—one week we went with Dad to the Episcopal Church and the next week to the Catholic Church with Mom. However, my Mom took me to CCD[39] and had me make my First Communion. When I was older, I chose to be confirmed as a Roman Catholic.

When I was growing up I heard talk about how Catholics and Protestants didn't get along, but I couldn't see any difference. Looking back, I definitely believed in God and Jesus, but I didn't have any sound reasons for choosing Catholicism over anything else. The differences I did see were in the quality of the music, the length of the service, and whether cookies were served after church—things that really had nothing to do with theology.

But in high school and especially in college, the more I learned about the Catholic faith, the more I came to love it. The thing that really confirmed my faith, however, was my required freshman theology course at Notre Dame with Father Groody. He encouraged us to doubt our faith and to question all things, large and small. He told us that parents don't encourage their children to question their faith because they're afraid they will lose it. He believed when you ask questions, you either lose your faith or it becomes a lot stronger. At the time, I thought, "This guy's crazy."

Then, in my sophomore year, I took Philosophy 101— another required course at Notre Dame—and we talked about all the big questions, such as what is time, what it means "to be," and what is a person. I loved this course and even though it was not a theology class, I started making all these connections in my head. Even if there is change in the world, something underlying must remain constant and, I realized, that is God. That's why He says "I AM"—He doesn't need to say more than that, He just is. Because of this course and the questions it posed, I started thinking philosophically about my faith and applying reason and logic for the first time.

I really like the logic of the Church, even though I don't fully understand it at this point in my life. When I was growing up I used to think that the Catholic Church was pretty old-fashioned. "Why doesn't it just get with the times?" I wondered. But it doesn't "just get with the times" because it thinks so profoundly. What seem like old-fashioned attitudes about issues like contraception and homo-sexuality are really the result of a deep understanding of the nature of human beings. For the Church to "get with the times" would be to deny the underlying truth. The Church is logical and consistent and that's important.

---

39. CCD or Confraternity of Christian Doctrine is the religious education program for children in the Catholic Church.

The sense of community that the Church provides is also really important to me. In college I took part in a weekly Bible study that included music, worship, and lectures. A lot of my friends had grown up in Christian communities and there was just a sense of family in our friendships. During senior year, I lived in an apartment off campus with two other girls. Every day we did morning prayer together and we got together for a couple of dinners every week as well. The way we shared our lives reminded me of the way the Apostles had shared their lives in common. Sometimes we disagreed, but I know you don't have to always agree with someone to support them in love on their Christian journey.

I have found strength in the Church community. One of my college roommates invited me to be a bridesmaid at her wedding in St. Louis. The day after the wedding, everyone attended Sunday Mass at the cathedral followed by a picnic in the park. I remember feeling so alive in that cathedral. There were people from the parish who were total strangers as well as the newlywed couple and people from the wedding, some of whom I knew and others whom I did not. We were all sharing the Eucharist. When I went up for Communion, Christ became a part of me and I became a part of Him and a part of all those other people around me. I thought of people around the world going to Mass and doing the same thing and I felt I was part of them and they were part of me. It is this universality that I love about the Church.

My choice of a medical school was difficult and went right down to the wire. I was accepted by several schools. To help me decide between them, I made spreadsheets to compare and contrast them. But, by the time finals ended and Senior Week began, the deadline was only days away and I still hadn't made up my mind which med school to choose. One of the big issues I was struggling with was cost. A private school like Tufts, which I liked, would cost $60,000, but a state school like the University of Massachusetts would be much more affordable. Everyone in the senior class wanted to go out and do fun things before graduation, but I just wanted to hole up by myself, to disappear for a couple of days, and to think about my decision. I guess what I needed was a retreat.

I finally went with a friend to her parents' house by a lake, taking my spreadsheets with me. In my prayer time I sat with my spreadsheets and asked God to help me, but I just didn't get any clear answer. My friend and I went for a walk along the beach; after talking with her, I was able to make a decision. I sat with it for a day and then decided the best choice for me was the University of Massachusetts.

But I deferred my acceptance to med school for a year so that I could spend time in Costa Rica as a volunteer in FrancisCorps, a small organization connected with the Franciscan friars. I lived with four other volunteers across the street from the Franciscan monastery. Each of us worked in a different part of the city. Half of our mission was our volunteer work; the other half was building a community together that was modeled on the way the friars lived. The community aspect was a huge reason why I chose this program as well, along with a desire to practice my Spanish.

I loved living in that kind of community and I loved my work, which was at a clinic in the capital city, San Jose. Originally the clinic was strictly a pediatric palliative care facility, but to meet the community's needs it had expanded its mission to include children with chronic illness and those with severe pain. The clinic's mission was to care not just for the child, but also for his or her whole family. When a child has great needs, the entire family suffers and needs support. Entire families came to the clinic in the morning with their children and they'd stay until about three in the afternoon. While they were there, they would see a doctor as well as a nurse, a physical therapist, a psychologist, and a nutritionist. Every staff member at the clinic was considered important, even the cook and the cleaning lady. They all worked together to care for these children and their families.

As part of a team of volunteers, my job was to plan social activities for the children while they waited to see the doctor and other staff members. I used to tell people I was a "professional spoiler" of children because that's what I did all day, every day. We colored pictures, played with trucks, and sang songs. I made up activities to correspond with the seasons and holidays. While I was playing with a child, the doctor might pull the child out of the activity for an exam, or the nutritionist might meet with the mother. The children were often tense. My job was to help them to relax and feel like normal kids for a day, despite their illness.

Working at the clinic was a good learning experience for me. I could see God everywhere. Since I was not a physician, I didn't do anything medically significant, but it was so powerful and important to talk to these children. Because they were there every day in my presence, I could tell them, "You're not different, you're not worthless. You have so much worth, so much dignity." The children were very needy, but so was I in a way. I have a desire to be needed. When other people need me I feel good. I realize that God used my desire to enable me to love the children in a special way.

People asked me if it was hard working in that clinic. In fact, it was easy because I enjoyed it and had great support from the Franciscan community. I began every day with prayer, giving each day completely to serving God. We knew that we were volunteers for Christ. Our job was to preach by our actions. Like St. Francis is said to have taught, "Preach the gospel every day; use words only if necessary." So, for example, I tried to preach by sitting next to a little boy who couldn't speak or move. At least I was there; I could read a book, sing a song, or tell silly stories to him. I never knew when it could be his last day with me, so I'd just spoil him as much as possible while I had him.

But as much as I love children, it was challenging to remain energetic around them day after day. Playing with the same truck for the eleventh time got old for me. But because it was new and exciting for the children, I had to be excited for them—I had to be the "professional spoiler" I was called to be. Because of the support of my faith community, I was able to return to the clinic fresh each day, to avoid treating it as a same-old, same-old job.

They say the Lord works in mysterious ways and it was true in my work at the clinic. On my application for the job, I gave myself high marks on some things, but not creativity. But somehow, mysteriously, I learned to be creative and came up with ways to entertain the children every day.

At every holiday I devised projects to celebrate the day. Of course they don't celebrate Thanksgiving in Costa Rica and because there is no winter, I couldn't design any snowman-related projects. But I learned to be creative and work around that. For example, nobody in Costa Rica knew who St. Patrick was, but I'm a good Domer[40], so by golly, when March rolled around, I announced that I was importing the holiday, and we had a huge St. Patrick's Day celebration. Notre Dame would have been so proud of me.

One interesting thing I learned is that kids cry for many reasons. Sometimes it's because their meds have worn off and they're in pain. Sometimes it's because a child misses their mom

---

40. A "Domer" is anyone affiliated with the University of Notre Dame. The golden dome with its 16-foot statue of the Blessed Virgin sits atop the historic main building on campus. The dome has become a symbol of the University.

and you're not her. That's such a human reason to cry. One day I sat with one girl who began crying when her mom went off to get a prescription filled. As I was wiping away her tears, I thought, "That's all I can do for her right now." But I felt like I was wiping away Christ's tears.

I also saw how universal the whole human experience is. Once I spent an entire day with a girl who couldn't walk. I didn't discover until a few days later, from someone's offhand remark, that she was also blind. When she came back later, the doctor asked her mom if she had any concerns beyond those of her daughter. The mom told him she was concerned about her older son because he played hooky every day instead of going to school. "What a universal issue," I thought, "This woman has a child with so many needs, who's blind and can't walk, yet she still worries about her son who won't go to school."

The clinic staff arranged for her son to work on a coffee plantation picking beans, so at least he could earn an income. I must have mentioned that I liked coffee, because a few weeks later, when the family returned to the clinic, the blind girl handed me a burlap-sack full of red things that looked like berries.

"What is this?" I asked the mother.

"It's coffee!" the girl piped up. "You said you liked coffee, so I told my brother he had to pick some coffee for you!" I thought, "Oh my gosh, she bosses her older brother around and she can't even walk!" Some family relationships are the same no matter what problems you have or where you live.

I had moments when I'd think, "Honestly, what good am I doing? I'm not a doctor, I'm not somebody's mom." Sometimes I felt like my presence just annoyed the kids. A lot of Costa Rican college students also volunteered at the clinic, so there were days when I felt I really didn't need to be there. But there were little moments of consolation, when I knew that my personal presence had made a difference in someone's life.

I spent one day with a boy who was about 15 years old. He could barely speak, but he had that typical teen-age way of saying nothing but still making fun of you through facial expressions and body language. We played video games and made a puzzle together and at the end of the day, his mother said to me, "Rebecca, I'm so glad you were with my son today. Some of the other volunteers don't know how to interact with him because he doesn't really talk and it's awkward. Because you played and joked around with him, you made him feel like he's no different from anyone else. You made him feel that he's special." Moments like that were good.

I also discovered in Costa Rica that I could be a lot more open about my faith and talk about it with people. I didn't have to ask permission to pray over a patient, like you have to do in the United States. The moms would pray for each other and ask us to pray for their children. They felt free to say things like, "It's a miracle my daughter is doing so well today." Even their everyday language acknowledged the presence of God. If you greeted someone with a "Good morning, how are you?" the standard response was "Fine, thank God." When you left and said "See you later," the response was "God willing"—literally, "If God wants it." This was true even for those who weren't religious. I really miss that in the United States. It seems that here, if you say the most mundane thing about religion, people start shaking or twitching.

After my year in Costa Rica, I began my studies in medical school at UMass—the University of Massachusetts in Worcester. Even though I had grown up in Massachusetts, I struggled with how secular and liberal it was. After four years at a Catholic university I guess I was shocked at the opinions and views of some of my classmates and professors. For example, we had a weekly small-group class to cover non-academic issues about being a doctor such as building relationships with and interviewing patients. An actor would portray the patient and one of the students would play the role of the doctor. Then we'd discuss and evaluate the conversation.

One week the subject was genetic counseling. The "patient" was pregnant and was nervous that her baby would have cystic fibrosis, since her nephew had suffered from that disease. She wasn't sure what she wanted to do about the pregnancy, whether to keep the child or have an abortion.

After the role-playing, the professor praised the med student's work in the interview with the patient. The professor noted that the student never called the baby a "baby." Because it was feared using the word "baby" would create emotional anxiety in the mother, it was always a fetus. Furthermore, the student never called the mother a "mother", or the father a "father" because neither had yet decided to be a parent. And, of course, the professor considered it important that the student had provided the patient with information about abortion options.

I just sat there and thought, "Oh, my gosh, I can't believe this." I know that many doctors use this approach; I know that some of my classmates are pro-choice. But I couldn't believe that my school would teach its students that they shouldn't do it any other way. To me that's just lying to the patient to make her feel better. Although I'm not out to make my patients cry, I believe that this approach provides false assurance and hides the truth from the patient.

Dealing with the secular atmosphere at UMass has been hard. At Notre Dame I had a really strong Catholic community and a strong support network of friends but when I came here I did not know anyone. At the beginning of my first year at UMass I joined a weekly Bible study, which has been a big help. The Worcester Guild of the Catholic Medical Association has also been a huge blessing for me. I found out about the Guild through the Diocese of Worcester's annual White Mass for health care professionals, which they celebrate each year at the St. Vincent Hospital chapel. Sometimes I feel lost and discouraged but it's great to have the support of these older and wiser Catholic doctors in the Guild. They show me that I can keep training to be a physician without giving up my faith. They help me believe I will make it and everything will be okay.

The Guild has been especially helpful to me with the issue of physicians' rights. These days our culture sees patient autonomy as the be-all and end-all. Politicians want to elevate patient autonomy so high that it takes away the rights of doctors to follow their own consciences. The doctors from the Guild are there to tell me "You don't have to do those things like abortions when you have moral objections. You don't even have to watch." The professors at UMass won't tell you that.

The Guild even brought in a lawyer last year to talk about the current state of the law on the subject of physicians' rights. She explained that the law does provide conscience protection, but that this is being threatened and could be lost. Honestly, I guess I just don't get it. I know I disagree with most of my classmates on certain points about what's harmful for the patient and what's not. I know my conscience tells me one thing and their consciences tell them something completely different. But don't we all have the right to follow our conscience?

My classmates know where I stand on certain things but I'm afraid of being labeled a "troublemaker." I got a little taste of that last year when I invited a Catholic physician from the Guild to give a guest lecture on natural family planning (NFP). I sent an email invitation to the entire school saying everyone was welcome to learn about this method of birth control as an option for patients who have religious, moral, or ecological issues with artificial birth control methods.

The next day a second-year student sent out a response—also to the entire school—attacking my statistics on the effectiveness of natural family planning. She cited an article filled with inaccuracies that lumped NFP in with the rhythm method and some other less reliable techniques. What she was really doing was calling me out in front of the entire school. It made me feel terrible. But one of my classmates stood up for me and, even though he was very busy, spent a lot of time looking up some more accurate data in support of NFP. The next morning he presented the data to the second-year student who had challenged me. Later he told me later he was angry with her for bashing me.

The lecture went really well and was well attended. Friends from my Bible study group came as well as students interested in alternative medicine who wanted to learn about NFP because it is a natural method of family planning that doesn't involve drugs. We actually had some pro-choice people attend the lecture. Two of them came up to me afterwards and thanked me for setting up the event. I was really surprised.

I finished my first year of med school in May and this past summer, I spent six weeks in Uganda through a grant from the Global Health Program administered though UMass. I was part of a team that developed a safe pregnancy/safe birth presentation. We traveled from village to village with an interpreter, presenting the program to pregnant women. Uganda has a high infant mortality rate; most women give birth at home and often don't use safe practices. Health care there is supposed to be free and universal, but the government of Uganda is pretty corrupt, and in practice this free care is not always available. We urged women to come to the clinics to give birth, but if that would be impossible, we also taught them how to have a safe birth at home.

Although the project was sponsored by a secular organization, my team leader was Christian and we became a huge support for each other. The rest of the team was doing this work for the good of humanity. We were there for that, of course, but also to serve Jesus.

My team leader had a connection to CURE International, a Christian organization with hospitals all over the world. One day she took us on a field trip to CURE's hospital in Uganda, which specialized in pediatric neurosurgery for patients with hydrocephalus. While we were there, I had some down time, so I wandered over to the waiting area to be with the moms and their children. I didn't speak any of their many dialects, but through signs I asked one of the mothers if I could hold her baby.

Although this baby had a huge head due to hydrocephalus, I sat there holding him like any normal baby. All the moms were so surprised because in Africa, many still believe that an illness like hydrocephalus is due to a curse on the baby or on the mother. But holding this child as I did was a non-verbal way for me to say, "This child deserves love like any other child, because that's the way God loves all children."

I'm really excited to know that one day I'll be a professional healer. I want to work in medical missions in developing countries. Unfortunately that's not a medical specialty so I still have to choose one. I'm leaning toward family medicine or pediatrics. Every time I go on a mission trip, such as the one to Uganda, my love for medicine is totally renewed. When I'm in a clinic and working with patients, I feel so alive. Being the presence of Christ for the sick and the needy is my dream. I hope I never lose that.

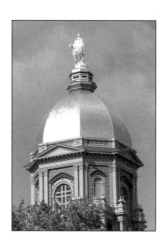

The dome at the University of Notre Dame.

— Ad Majorem Dei Gloriam —

12

Dr. James Walsh

A SUBTLE THING

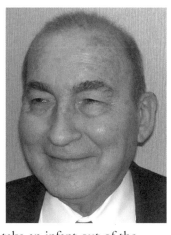

I was born in 1930 and baptized into the Catholic Church as a baby. My parents were both Irish Catholic, and in those days we were all baptized when we were a week old, because you didn't dare take an infant out of the house before it was baptized. I was raised in Waterbury, Connecticut where my parents moved after they were married. My father was a typewriter salesman for most of my early life. He was a 20-year veteran of the Army, served in both World War I and World War II, and was on active duty in the Army Reserves during the Korean War. I had four other brothers and sisters; I was the middle child. I was brought up by my parents in an atmosphere in which we tried to practice good sense and keep our religion as well as we could.

My family was never overly involved in parish life, but we went to church regularly for Mass and for Sunday afternoon benediction. I was an altar server for a while. I attended St. Margaret Parochial School and Sacred Heart High School. Grammar school was rather unexciting, though high school was good. Though a small school with rather primitive facilities, Sacred Heart had good academics and a strong athletic program. I was never an athlete, but I followed the school sports closely and was manager of the basketball team.

After Sacred Heart I went to the College of the Holy Cross here in Worcester. My older brother had gone to Holy Cross for about a year and then went into the seminary and I just kind of followed along behind him. I'm sure it was difficult financially for my parents to pay for college for both of us, but you'd never know it because they never made an issue out of it. Of course I had a partial scholarship and college wasn't as expensive in 1948 as it is now. After my first year at Holy Cross, I applied to go into the seminary, as my brother had. I was accepted to a seminary down in

Connecticut but I never did attend. I'm not sure what happened; I just never followed up with it, and by the time September rolled around I decided to go back to Holy Cross after all.

At Holy Cross we had four years of theology and philosophy; we were taught the things a true Catholic college should teach. You can't help but be affected by that. I majored in mathematics and pre-med. It was a heavy load of courses. I took pre-med mainly because it was a good course of study even though at that time I wasn't yet interested in becoming a doctor. In fact, I wasn't enthused about medicine till senior year. Why did I become interested in medicine? It's a strange thing, but I have no idea.

I attended medical school at Georgetown University in Washington, DC. I enjoyed my four years there but it was hard work. I made some good friends with whom I've kept in touch over the years, especially a group of six students from freshman year anatomy class with whom I did dissection. I had no clear idea of what I wanted to specialize in when I finished med school and so I went on to do a general internship in Worcester at St. Vincent Hospital. After my internship I thought I might go into neurology, but I was drafted into service in the Army. That was in 1957 and although the Korean War was over, unless you had committed yourself to something else as a doctor, you had to serve in the Army. I went for basic training in Texas and within three months I was in Korea.

I spent 15 months with the Army in Korea. Most of my deployment was spent with a group of 10 or 12 Americans serving as an advisory group at the headquarters for the training of the South Korean army. This detachment usually didn't have a doctor, because there was no great necessity for one. The place was very isolated and there wasn't much to do. But it was interesting in its own way, and I enjoyed my time there. We treated sick and injured Americans and acted as medical advisors to the Koreans who staffed the nearby hospital. We always had to rely on translators, because I didn't speak Korean in those days and neither did the rest of the Army personnel. Our unit was one of several small groups stationed in different places, attached to the Korean army. When the doctor for one of the other units was sick or away, I would be assigned to go there and fill in. That's where I met some of the missionary groups who were working in Korea.

One group I met was the Brothers of St. John of God, a nursing order from Ireland. They ran a general clinic in the southern city of Gwangju that offered treatment for all kinds of diseases. I got to know some of the missionaries pretty well. After my discharge from the Army Father Richers came to visit to ask if I'd think of going back to Korea as a missionary. It seemed that the brothers had a doctor who was leaving in six months and they needed someone to replace him. So I finished up my general medical training at St. Vincent and went back to work in Korea for the next four years.

I worked with five religious brothers, all of whom were registered nurses. We saw every medical problem under the sun. Eventually an x-ray technician joined us. The technician was especially welcome because we saw a lot of tuberculosis and pneumonia. Before the x-ray technician came, we would have to send patients elsewhere for x-rays, and sometimes they wouldn't return for treatment. Subsequently, one of the brothers trained as a doctor and joined our mission. There were a number of religious orders working in Korea at the time I was there: the Columban Fathers, the Columban Sisters, the Brothers of St. John of God, the Maryknolls, Mother Seton's Sisters of Charity, and the Caritas Sisters. Nowadays, some of the religious from Korea are coming to the United States to serve here.

Korea is one of the few countries that were converted to Christianity from within. I have in my office a small statue of St. Andrew Kim, the first Korean martyr. He was one of several Koreans in the 1800s who, having heard stories about Christianity, traveled to China to learn more about it. He converted to the Faith, was ordained a priest, and returned to proselytize his own people. Kim was only back in Korea a few months when he was murdered because of his Christian faith. Pope John Paul II canonized him in 1984.

In the days when I was there, Korea was primitive, medically speaking. We saw anywhere between 100 and 200 patients a day, with all kinds of diseases—the kinds you'd see here now in the United States, plus many others that we might have seen here 100 years ago. The patients included a large number of people with tuberculosis and many people suffering from malnutrition.

I particularly remember twin girls who were very malnourished. The girls' mother was working, trying to provide for her children, but was unable to take care of them. Their feet were terribly deformed, twisted inward, and we knew that without treatment they would never walk. In those days, a problem like that often went untreated in Korea.

We didn't have an orthopedic specialist, but we were able to pay a Korean doctor to come and take care of the children. It wasn't a question of doing surgery, but rather of putting casts on their feet and recasting them frequently as they grew. In fact, the first casts fell off because the girls were so thin. Eventually, though, the doctor was able to straighten out their feet and their legs became perfectly normal. The twins grew up very nicely and both entered the convent. Years later when I would go back to visit Korea, I would often see them.

We saw a few lepers too. We had to keep them separated from the other patients because the Koreans, like most people, were afraid of catching leprosy. In those days we didn't have much to treat the leprosy itself, but we took care of their other problems: sore throat, pneumonia, that sort of thing. We had to be careful, because once people found out we were treating lepers, they wouldn't come to our clinic. The other problem was that the Koreans (like all of us, I suppose) expected quick treatments and results. A lot of patients wouldn't come back if you didn't cure them right away, and of course you can't cure leprosy quickly. Leprosy still can't be cured completely, but today there are treatments that make the disease non-infectious, so leprosy doesn't have the stigma it once had.

Some of the brothers I worked with were pretty memorable. Brother Bede, who was from Ireland, was a real character. The Koreans loved him because he was always joking and he made them happy even when they had problems—and most of the people we saw had big problems. Once a patient came to Brother Bede and asked him where the toilet was. The bathrooms in those days were outhouses a good distance behind the clinic. Brother Bede pointed them out to the patient and joked, "Why don't you wait ten minutes, and the bus will take you down there." One of the others, Brother Brendon, had a thick Irish accent and I had a tough time understanding him. When I mentioned this to Brother Bede, he smiled and told me, "Don't worry. We don't understand him either."

As time went on, the brothers opened up a beggars' camp to care for the medical needs of the community's beggars, who until then were not getting help from anybody. Later they opened up a psychiatric hospital, which became the main part of their mission. Three of four of the Irish brothers still work there, but primarily Korean brothers are doing the work now.

It was very easy for me to keep my faith when I was in Korea. I lived in the monastery for the first three of my four years there, until a separate house was built for the doctors. My room was right across from the chapel and often I would participate in the community's prayers.

I was in Korea for four years, but since then, I've gone back four or five times to visit the community and the clinic. The last time I went was this past November, when the community celebrated its 50th anniversary. They were also celebrating the ordination of two new priests, both of them Korean. It was a big event for them—these were the first two Koreans to be ordained in the order. Most of the members of the community are just brothers, not priests. They aren't near enough to any other religious community where a priest could say Mass for them every day, so this was a great milestone for them. While I was there, I met up with a Korean nurse whom I hadn't seen since I left Gwangju in 1966. It was a great time.

Most of the brothers are Korean now—there are just three Irishmen remaining. One of them came to Korea the year after I did, and though in his 80s, he's still busy in the community. He "retired" a number of years ago and went back to Ireland, but he found he couldn't stand it and returned. He'd been in Korea so long, I guess he was used to the weather! So he finally went back, and he's been there for over 20 years now. He's working in a home for the aged and mentally ill, feeding and caring for the patients. The community now has two or three different houses and a psychiatric hospital, which were built after I left. Br. Brendon is the only one of the original group of brothers still alive.

Friendship was not the only thing that kept me connected with the Korean mission. A group of doctors and nurses here in Worcester had started an organization to collect and sort samples of medicines and send them to Korea for our clinic. After I finished my time in Korea, I felt that if I didn't get involved with the project, it would probably disappear. So I continued the medical collections. Eventually as Korea became more modern and developed its own drug firms, our donations were no longer needed.

When I returned from Korea in 1966, I started my own practice in internal medicine in downtown Worcester. I moved into this office when the building was constructed in 1974. Much has changed in medicine since that time. The treatments have improved for things like infectious diseases that you couldn't cure before.

Cardiology today is great; cardiac surgery is marvelous. They're doing so much in cancer surgery too—they can detect it so early and can treat it medically or surgically. I remember when patients who had eye surgery used to have to lie in bed for days, with pillows propped all around so they wouldn't move their heads. Well, now, my God, the patients go home that day and the next day they see perfectly!

The *way* medicine is practiced has also changed a lot too, although not necessarily for the better. I've had a solo practice for most of my career. Now I think that solo practice—what is called today primary care—is kind of dying out. The government makes it so difficult—the amount of paperwork means that you never get the work done. And some of that paperwork is stupid. If I send you to a specialist and he orders certain tests for you, I'd probably be the one who has to explain why the tests were needed, even though I didn't order them. The bureaucracy is just terrible.

You have to pray all the time, because medicine can be tough. You may have problems finding a diagnosis for a patient, or dealing with a difficult person who's testy about everything. You have to ask God to help you with those things, even if sometimes it doesn't seem to help. I had a priest-confessor one time who told me to be patient with my patients. I said, "Yeah, Father, that's easy for you to say!" But you try to take that advice and ask God to help you to control your temper, especially when you walk into work the next day and you have four or five of the kinds of patients who make you want to strangle them. I'm talking about people who are taking too many pills and are after you all the time for more. It's your job as a doctor to try to control that and keep them from getting hooked. But it can be very difficult. Some of those patients can be very persistent and devious, like the woman who keeps calling to ask for a new prescription. She says her prescription was stolen from her purse, yet the wallet the prescription was in was not taken! That doesn't seem likely.

I try not to preach, really. I try to help as much as I can. But I'm sure sometimes I end up preaching anyway even though I don't realize it when I start. But people are funny—you can't really preach to them and have the effect you want.

My patients range in age from 20 to over 100 years old. Just two days ago I saw a nun who is 102. She's ailing but at 102, we all slow down! She uses a cane but she's got all her marbles. Last year, at 101 years old, she wrote a book. I can't remember the topic; it was something to do with Catholic spirituality. She dresses as I think a nun should dress, with the veil and wimple and whatnot. It's a pleasure to have her in my office. I try to remember patients like her to help me overcome my irritation with the ones who pester me. Most of the time with my older patients, I talk about things that don't have to do with health at all. I'll be sitting with them and then we will go off on tangents and I'll realize, "What am I doing? We haven't talked about any of his medical problems. Get back on track!"

It's hard to explain how Catholic faith affects my medical practice. It fits in with your whole life really, in a subtle way. You have a basic set of moral principles that you try to follow, and I think following them makes you a better doctor.

I've had some patients who have inspired me, especially grown children who sacrifice a lot for their parents. Some people put their elderly parents in a nursing home, but a lot of people still care for them at home. I've had cases where one of the children has given up his job to take over the parent's care. The other siblings and family members help out financially so that, in the end, the whole family helps out in one way or another. It impresses me a lot when people do things like that, especially because it's a struggle that can last years and years.

In my own family's case, we were very lucky; my parents were very well almost to the day they died. My father died suddenly of a heart attack on the day before I was supposed to go to Korea, on the feast of St. John of God. My mother lived alone and we all took care of her, but she was a very independent woman—she drove and everything till she was 91 years old. When she was 92, she became ill with hepatitis (we never knew from what), was in the hospital, and then sent for short-term rehab. She died a week later.

I'm one of the team physicians for the College of the Holy Cross athletic teams. I usually attend the football and basketball games and travel with the basketball team to four or five away games a year. These are usually day or overnight trips so I use them as mini-vacations. I'm not the type to go away for two weeks to a beach somewhere—that would drive me crazy! I'm there at the games in case of emergency. The teams also have two orthopedic surgeons, and the football team always takes at least one with them to the away games, because orthopedic injuries are common. Of course with an injury that's serious (and we've had some), you get the player off to the hospital.

I have a lot of religious art in my office. My favorite piece is a Pieta by Guiseppi Armani. It has a very Baroque look to it, with figures with swirling hair and capes. The artist is still alive— I have several of his pieces. I also have a statue of the Korean St. Andrew Kim; he's boldly holding the Cross. And I have a figure that resembles the posture of Rodin's *Thinker*, but instead, it's a monk contemplating a skull. Does the artwork help me in my prayer life? It may, I suppose; I don't know. If it does, it's a subtle thing. I just like it.

Modern art leaves me cold. I look at it and say, "What does that mean?" But even religious art can be horrible. Some of it is just gaudy, even though I'm sure the artists mean well. One time someone gave me a religious painting that was a family heirloom. It was awful! I felt like throwing it away, but I thought, "I can't. It's someone's family treasure." I think I still have it in my basement.

On my wall I have copy of *The Physician's Prayer* and of Pope John Paul II's millennial declaration, along with a pro-life declaration signed by President Ronald Reagan. And there's also a photograph of me with Eileen Farrell, my favorite opera singer, whom I once met at the Metropolitan Opera in New York. I had the opportunity to visit her and her family in their apartment and she even gave me copies of a few of her private recordings. The photograph was taken when I was sent to see her off at the airport. She was a great singer, with a powerful voice. I'm a founding member of Opera Worcester; I've been treasurer and president at various times and I'm still on the board. I'm the only founding member left.

I got used to going to daily Mass back in college at Holy Cross. In those days, attendance at daily Mass was required. Since then I've continued. I'm not overt about it—it's a subtle thing. If I don't start off the day with Mass, I feel kind of lost in a way. Daily Mass affects my whole purpose and way of doing things.

I've been involved in a lot of pro-life work. I help support Visitation House, a home for unwed mothers on Endicott Street in Worcester. I'm on the board of Problem Pregnancy, which has an office across from the Planned Parenthood abortion clinic. Problem Pregnancy does sidewalk counseling and holds prayer vigils outside of the abortion clinic. I used to do that too, but not in a number of years.

I never felt a "calling" to the single life per se, but circum-stances were such that I just never got around to marriage. In a sense, the single life is a selfish life; after a number of years you get used to doing things your own way. You can come and go when you please, and you have no one to tell you that you can't do this or can't do that. When you marry, you have to bend your ways a bit. To get married late in life, I think, is crazy. A single person always misses having a family, but sometimes you're so busy you don't think of that.

It's hard to juggle a family and a medical practice. You can't be selfish if you have a family. It's true you have your practice, which is very important, but I won't say it comes first. Anybody who marries a doctor has got to be very patient, very understanding. But you can't ignore your family and I think a lot of doctors end up doing that. They don't mean to do it, but they get so entranced with their practice and their medical life that they tend to ignore their families, which is not good. A family needs attention. I think that's also one of the many reasons why priests should not marry. They just wouldn't be able to concentrate on their primary job, which is taking care of their parishioners.

An upbringing in the Faith does make you a little more sympathetic to people's problems, and it also prompts you to try to help in a spiritual sense. You do have to be careful talking about religion with patients; you should make sure you know what they're thinking first. It can be difficult, especially with someone who hasn't gone to church in a long time. But it's not impossible. Of course, not all my patients are Catholic. But while I do worry about their physical problems—that's my job as a doctor—I try to remember that every patient also has spiritual needs. If one of my Catholic patients is seriously ill or in the emergency room, I try to always make sure that a priest is called. That's especially true if I know the patient is dying or could possibly die. Fortunately, at St. Vincent Hospital, where I practice, a priest is always available. I can let him know if I'm aware that the patient has some problem with their faith, so the priest can do his job and help get things straightened out.

I had a situation like that in my own family. My brother had been away from the Church for many years. He had been married twice, and his second marriage was outside the Church. When he was dying in Walter Reed Medical Center, I called the hospital's chaplain to explain that my brother was baptized a Catholic but I had no idea what his situation was in terms of his faith. I wanted the priest to visit my brother so he could set things right with God if he needed to do that before he died. To my surprise, when I reached the chaplain, he told me he'd already seen my brother. "That's all taken care of," he said.

I think the end-of-life issues will be studied, argued about, and complained about as time goes on. We're getting older and living longer. I see patients who tell me their age, and I ask them, "You're *how* old? You're not that old!" Older people are more active today, leading "productive" lives, whatever that means. Some of them are still working at jobs. I had one patient who was 82 years old with an artificial leg, but she was still working in a small factory. Her boss used to pick her up every day to bring her to work because she was such a good employee. So you can't put anybody in categories based on age.

And I'm sure obstetricians meet up with a lot of problems connected with the beginning of life, especially when it comes to couples who want a child and can't have one. The medical world goes to great lengths in cases like that, with Petri dishes and all this other business. I vividly remember a couple who went to med school with me—I think they're both Catholic, in fact I'm sure of it. They were telling me about their grandchild who had been conceived that way, going on and on about this wonderful child. Well, I said to myself (because I knew I wasn't going to convince *them*) "That ain't the way to do it." It's ironic that people are killing babies all the time; yet other people are so desperate to have a child they go about it the wrong way.

I see medicine as a vocation. Medicine is a vocation even if you're not Catholic, but I think it helps to be Catholic. You have to have certain moral principles that you're going to apply to whatever you do. It's kind of an unconscious thing, but it's there. The Catholic faith helps you to look at the patient as not just another patient, but in a certain sense, as another Christ. It's like our call to help the beggar down the street. People will say, "He's a fake" or whatever, and they may be right. But we have to remember, there are stories in the Bible about situations like that, where Christ appears in a form we don't expect. And even if it's not Christ, that beggar is a creature of God, Who created us all. We're all equal in His eyes. He loves us all—that's the strange thing. Why He does, I don't know! So we should love one another, even if it's sometimes hard to do. If you help the beggar, you will be rewarded, even if that guy is a fake. That's the same way physicians should approach their patients to help them. It's hard to explain, but I think being a faithful Catholic makes you a better doctor.

But times are changing. Doctors thought differently 20 or 30 years ago. When St. Vincent Hospital wanted to close its obstetrical unit, it was the doctors who rose up. The hospital was perfectly willing to let it go, but we told them why they shouldn't, from a religious standpoint. And of course the OB unit is still in existence now. Nowadays the medical staff is more diverse. You don't know the doctors at the hospital and even if they were Catholic, you wouldn't know it. Not that they're not good people, but there isn't a sense of the spiritual life as there used to be. In the old days, you knew the doctors were Catholic; not necessarily holy-holies, who carried something that said, "I'm Catholic" around their necks, but you knew their faith permeated their lives.

St. Vincent Hospital used to be run by the Sisters of Providence. Now a corporate hospital chain owns it. When I started, 60 nuns from that order were working there; now there's only one left—Sr. Mary O'Leary who's in her 80s but still working. But there's still a Catholic identity at St. Vincent. I believe there must have been something in the contract about that when the corporation bought the hospital. The hospital has a Catholic chapel and two chaplains on staff. The head chaplain, Monsignor Peter Beaulieu, has done a lot to keep the hospital's Catholic presence alive. He and I are good friends—we get together for lunch almost every day of the week in the cafeteria. Fortunately, the hospital president is a Catholic who is well aware of his faith. He has tried to reinforce the Catholic identity of the institution. He did that because of his own faith, but I think it's a smart move too, because a lot of people in the community go there because it is a Catholic hospital.

Here in Massachusetts I'm active in the Worcester Guild of the Catholic Medical Association. Our meetings are pretty interesting—sometimes Monsignor Peter, the hospital head chaplain, speaks to us about medical and spiritual topics. I really wish we'd had an active CMA guild around here years ago. I've been to a couple of the national meetings of the association, and they're great, really enjoyable. The days are filled with lectures and talks and presentations, and we have daily Mass. It's kind of embarrassing in the sense that you meet people there who are doing all kinds of wonderful things, and it makes you think, "What have *I* done?" But even so, it's nice to talk with doctors who think just like you do.

Some of the CMA members have been very active in the public forum. I remember meeting one physician from Oregon who was leading the fight there against physician-assisted suicide. That's another big problem that's going to become more prominent in the coming years. I just can't understand how doctors can get involved in something like that, but they do. And the sad thing is that so many of these patients are not really dying of something terrible, even though they are sick. A few autopsies of assisted-suicide patients have shown nothing at all. The patient just wanted to die. When I was training in med school, not even the secular doctors would think of doing such a thing.

That's why we need an organization like the Catholic Medical Association. These problems—abortion, end of life issues, doctors' rights of conscience—are getting worse and worse. You've got to fight these things tooth and nail, and one doctor cannot do it alone. And the regular medical societies aren't doing it, because like our society, they've become so secularized. In a way, Catholic doctors need to be the conscience for the medical profession. In the future I think the CMA is going to play a bigger role than ever, because it is the only group that has some stability in its thinking. The CMA can really help those doctors who say they don't believe in such-and-such procedure, but feel they have to go with the flow because everybody else thinks it's okay.

And that's true even for non-moral issues having to do with medicine. People always say that doctors stick together, but actually they don't—they're too independent. Some of the organizations that want to control health care have no idea of what it's like to be in a doctor's office—none. An individual doctor cannot fight these problems; it's like a voice crying in the wilderness. But if you have more than one voice, you might be able to do something. That's why the CMA is very important.

This year I'll turn 80. At the moment I have prostate cancer. I was on chemo for a while. The first treatment worked all right; the second did nothing. The third treatment helped for a while, but now it's failing and my PSA is up. The tumor has invaded the right ureter and I've had a couple of stents put in. My urologist wants me to go to a specialist in Boston, and I will go, but just to get another opinion and to see what they have to say about it. I refuse to go back and forth to Boston for treatment—that's crazy.

I'm still practicing medicine; it's been 54 years now, but it's a struggle—not because of pain, because I don't have pain, thank God. I'm just weak all the time, so weak that I have a tough time keeping up. I have my patients to see in the office and the hospital and I visit a lot of nursing homes. At one point I was seeing patients in 28 nursing homes. It can be very busy here, especially on Mondays, and I get so tired all the time. I've more or less decided that I'd better quit on July 1.

Our job as doctors is to try to relieve suffering, whether physical, mental or otherwise. You do your best to help. Sometimes it works and sometimes it doesn't. But when you can do nothing more, you can maybe try to encourage your patients to offer up their suffering.[41] We should do that, but we don't always—at least most of us don't. "Offering it up" is something we're just not tuned in to do. And it's difficult to get people in the mood to offer up their suffering. We want quick cures. We don't want to suffer. But of course, we're going to have to, whether we like it or not. That's the way life is.

Facing death should, in a certain way, affect our relationship with God. I know people who say, "I want to go just like *that*. I don't want to suffer for years." Well, I'm sorry, but I *don't* want to go just like that. I'm not one of those enthusiasts for sudden death. I don't necessarily want to suffer either, but it wouldn't hurt a person to suffer a little bit. I try hard, but I don't think I know any person who is suddenly just going to leap up to heaven when they die—myself included. I just hope I can leap into purgatory and work my way up from there.

Knowing you might die in a few years makes you try to be a little more attentive to the things you should be doing to prepare. We should always do that, of course, but it doesn't always work out that way. Human nature being what it is, we get distracted by everything around us, especially if we're young—which I'm not anymore. For young people, death is the last thing they ever think about, which makes it so tragic when you see people die young. Sudden death, especially, is a terrible thing to happen, and it makes you just worry that the person wasn't able to make peace with God beforehand.

Sometimes tragedy tests people's faith. They ask, "Why did God let this young person get cancer?" But none of us really knows why people get sick. We're all going to die someday. Some die

---

41. For an excellent discussion of redemptive suffering and the practice of "offering it up" see: http://www.fisheaters.com/offeringitup.html.

young; some die old. It has nothing to do with whether we're good or bad. It happens according to God's plan, and we don't know what that plan is. But seeing tragedy, even after all these years, hasn't really tested my faith. It would take far more than that to test it.

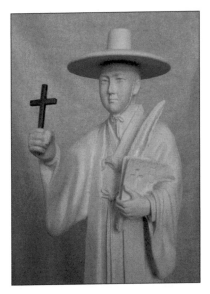

Dr. Walsh's statue of St. Andrew Kim of Korea

— Ad Majorem Dei Gloriam —

In Memoriam

On July 17th, 2010 Dr. James Walsh passed on from this life and went home to God. He spent his last days at the home of his sister, Anne. Many family members and friends came to visit him, including Brother Brendon of the Brothers of St. John of God with whom Dr. Walsh had served in Korea. The visits were exhausting for him, but full of laughter and joy. Each day Dr. Walsh received a tiny piece of the Eucharist. His funeral Mass took place in St. Paul's Cathedral in Worcester. Dr. Walsh was buried in the religious habit of the Brothers. Shortly before his death, in gratitude for his commitment and dedication, the Superior General of the Order made Dr. Walsh an affiliated member and permitted him to be buried in the habit of professed brothers.

POSTSCRIPT

Put on your stethoscope.
Listen slowly,
With more than your usual care.
Yet not to the heart of another,
Today to the sounds of your own.
What sounds, deep within your chest?
Abandon the chatter, be still and listen.

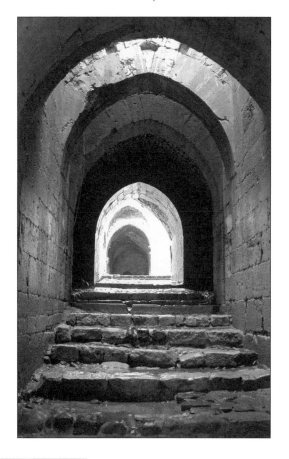

42. Photo: Krak des Chevaliers, Syria. Used courtesy of the Australian National University.

INDEX